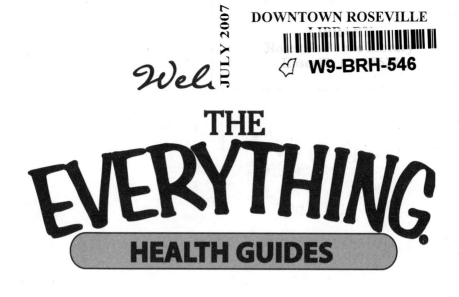

THE EVERYTHING

HEALTH GUIDES

W**hen you're faced** with a pressing health issue, your first instinct is to find out as much about it as you can. With so much conflicting information out there, where can you turn for professional, supportive advice?

Packed with the most recent, up-to-date data, THE EVERYTHING® HEALTH GUIDES help ensure that you get a good diagnosis, choose the best doctor, and find the right medical treatment. With this one comprehensive resource, you and your family members have all the information you could possibly need—at your fingertips.

THE EVERYTHING® HEALTH GUIDES are an extension of the best-selling Everything® series in the health category, which also includes *The Everything® Diabetes Book* and *The Everything® Menopause Book*. Accessible and easy to read, THE EVERYTHING® HEALTH GUIDES provide specific details and clear examples that relate to your given medical situation. If you're looking for one-stop, all-inclusive guides that allow you to understand and become more in tune with your body, this groundbreaking series is the perfect tool for you.

Visit the entire Everything® series at *www.everything.com*

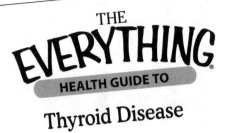

THE EVERYTHING

HEALTH GUIDE TO

Thyroid Disease

Dear Reader,

Chances are, you picked up this book because you or someone you care about has a thyroid condition. Or perhaps you're starting to suspect that you might have one. Maybe you can't understand why you can't ditch the weight despite your most noble efforts. Or maybe you're feeling inexplicably fatigued, depressed, or irritable.

In any case, this book is written for you—anyone who is trying to better understand the thyroid, how it functions when you're healthy, and what goes wrong when it becomes diseased. It's hard to imagine that a tiny gland nestled in your neck can have such power over the way you feel, how much you weigh, and even the texture of your skin and hair. But that's what the thyroid gland is—an anatomical powerhouse with enormous influence over your health and well-being.

We know it's not easy to live with a thyroid condition. Dr. Friedman has treated hundreds of patients with all sorts of thyroid disease and lived with Hashimoto's himself for several years. But we also know that having thyroid disease is not the end of the world. By the time you finish this book, we think you'll agree.

Sincerely,

Theodore C. Friedman, M.D., Ph.D.

Winnie Yu

THE
EVERYTHING

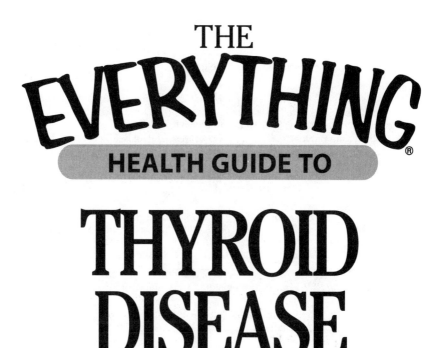

HEALTH GUIDE TO

THYROID
DISEASE

Professional advice on getting the
right diagnosis, managing your
symptoms, and feeling great

Theodore C. Friedman, M.D., Ph.D., and Winnie Yu

Adams Media
Avon, Massachusetts

Dedication

To my wonderful wife, Danielle, and my great kids,
Nora, Caleb, and Gideon.—T. F.
To Bill Glavin and John Keats for the early vote of confidence.—W. Y.

• • •

Publishing Director: Gary M. Krebs
Associate Managing Editor: Laura M. Daly
Associate Copy Chief: Brett Palana-Shanahan
Acquisitions Editor: Kate Burgo
Development Editor: Katie McDonough
Associate Production Editor: Casey Ebert

Director of Manufacturing: Susan Beale
Associate Director of Production:
Michelle Roy Kelly
Cover Design: Paul Beatrice, Erick DaCosta,
Matt LeBlanc
Layout and Graphics: Heather Barrett,
Brewster Brownville, Colleen Cunningham,
Jennifer Oliveira

An Everything® Series Book.
Everything® and everything.com® are registered trademarks of F+W Publications, Inc.

Published by Adams Media, an F+W Publications Company
57 Littlefield Street, Avon, MA 02322 U.S.A.
www.adamsmedia.com

ISBN 10: 1-59337-719-3
ISBN 13: 978-1-59337-719-9

Printed in the United States of America.

J I H G F E D C B A

Library of Congress Cataloging-in-Publication Data
Friedman, Theodore C.
The everything health guide to thyroid disease / Theodore C. Friedman and Winnie Yu.
p. cm. -- (An everything series book)
Includes index.
ISBN-13: 978-1-59337-719-9
ISBN-10: 1-59337-719-3
1. Thyroid gland--Diseases--Popular works. I. Yu, Winnie. II. Title.

RC655.F75 2007
616.4'4--dc22
2006028189

This book is available at quantity discounts for bulk purchases.
For information, please call 1-800-289-0963.

*All the examples and dialogues used in this book are fictional and have
been created by the author to illustrate possible situations.*

Acknowledgments

I'd like to thank my parents, Paula and Jeremy Hutt and Paul and Mona Friedman, for their love. I'd like to thank my clinic assistants, Dr. Erik Zuckerbraun, Claudia Murphy, Lynne Drabkowski, and Kimberly Daigle, for all their help with my patients. I thank my patients for teaching me about thyroid problems and encouraging me to think outside the box.

—*T. F.*

Most books don't come into existence without a strong supporting cast, and this one is no exception. I'd like to thank my editor, Kate Burgo, for her support; my collaborator, Dr. Ted Friedman, for his enthusiasm and steadfast guidance; and Mary J. Shomon for pointing the way. I'd also like to thank Doug Brunk, Jane Porter, Mary Jane Farney, Beth McNassor, Candy Hammond, Pat van derHeijden, and Susan Livada, who shared their personal experiences with thyroid disease with me. And, of course, I must thank Jeff, Samantha, and Annie, whose hugs and kisses get me through anything and everything.

—*W. Y.*

Contents

Introduction

These days, we hear so much about diabetes and heart disease—the rising incidence of both and the terrible toll they're taking on our nation's health and economy. But there's another condition that affects even more Americans: thyroid disease. The problem is, many people don't even know they have it.

According to the American Association of Clinical Endocrinologists, there are 27 million people in this country with some form of thyroid disease. Approximately half are unaware. But before you shrug it off as being less serious than heart disease or less bothersome than diabetes, consider this: having thyroid disease actually elevates your risk for both heart disease and diabetes. Those are just two reasons why thyroid health is so important.

Having a healthy thyroid has numerous implications for your life, your health, and your happiness. A healthy thyroid makes it easier for you to maintain your body weight, keeps depression at bay, and gives your cells the energy they need for all the activities you do. The proper amount of thyroid hormone is also essential for menstrual regularity, pregnancy, and the delivery of a healthy baby. An unhealthy thyroid, on the other hand, can cause problems as diverse as dry hair, difficulty concentrating, and muscle aches. It can make you perpetually uneasy, constantly exhausted, and sweaty for no good reason. In short, the thyroid gland affects virtually every aspect of your health and well-being.

That said, you may wonder how anyone could have a thyroid problem and not know it. It's simple. Many people with thyroid disease are being treated for their symptoms instead, especially if their TSH levels are only borderline abnormal. So rather than being properly treated for a thyroid problem, they're being given remedies for specific symptoms. An antidepressant for depression. A sleeping pill for insomnia. Stool softeners for constipation. For many people, treatment for the underlying thyroid disorder could correct all these symptoms—and even some that you might not know are associated with thyroid disease, such as high cholesterol.

That's why this book is so vital. Here, you will find the information, guidance, and strategies you need to get properly diagnosed and treated. You'll also learn the pitfalls of untreated thyroid disease and the perks of getting your thyroid condition under control.

By reading this book, you will glean the basic medical knowledge you need to talk intelligently with your doctor about your thyroid condition, so that you can ask smart questions, get the right tests, and get the appropriate treatments. More specifically, you will learn to distinguish a nodule from a goiter, a thyroid problem from postpartum depression, and hyperthyroidism from panic disorder. Best of all, you will do all this without wading through heavy medical terminology.

As you may already know, learning to deal with a thyroid condition—or any health problem for that matter—takes time, patience, and practice. At first, you may be frustrated by all the uncertainty as you try to determine whether you even have a thyroid problem. Then you have to wait for the medication to kick in or for the date of your radioactive iodine treatment to come, all the while still coping with the aggravating symptoms. Once you're treated, you may still have problems with your weight or experience recurrent symptoms or even new ones. All medical conditions come with their share of frustrations, and thyroid disease is no exception.

No, it's not always easy to have a thyroid disorder. But the good news about thyroid disease is that most people are readily treated and go on to live perfectly normal, healthy lives. The key to getting well and staying well is knowledge. You need to know what to do in order to be healthy. By picking up this book, you've made a commitment to learn as much as you can about your thyroid. And that's one giant first step toward better health.

All about Your Thyroid

Most of us don't give much thought to our thyroid glands. After all, a healthy thyroid doesn't really make its presence known. But in the scheme of the human body, this tiny gland is a vital part of our health and well-being. Sadly, it usually isn't until it malfunctions and causes disease that the thyroid gets any attention. This chapter offers an introduction to this great gland and all that it does for you.

A Busy Gland

Ever wonder why your best friend can down desserts with reckless abandon and never gain weight? And why you pack on pounds by nibbling on just one or two desserts a week? At least some of the blame—or credit, depending on whom you ask—goes to your thyroid, which produces the hormone that determines your metabolism, or basal metabolic rate (BMR). That's the rate at which your body cells use oxygen and energy to do their jobs. Too much thyroid hormone, and your metabolism speeds up. Too little, and it slows down.

But metabolic rate is only one of the thyroid gland's tasks. It is also responsible for how your body uses the energy sources—carbohydrates, proteins, and fats—that you derive from food. It is responsible for bone growth and muscle function. In addition, the thyroid affects respiration, heart rate, mood, skin, hair, and nails.

For all it does, the thyroid is a modest organ that weighs about half to three-quarters of an ounce in mature adults. On the body, the small butterfly-shaped gland resembles a bowtie, nestled in the front of your neck, just below the larynx—also called your Adam's apple or voice box—and in front of the trachea, the windpipe that carries air to your lungs. The wings of the butterfly are called its left and right lobes, and are wrapped around the trachea. Each lobe measures about an inch and a half. In between is the isthmus, a narrow strip that connects the two wings.

Alert

A drop in thyroid hormone can cause depression, malaise, and forgetfulness. An increase in thyroid hormone can cause excitability, wide fluctuations in mood, and crying spells for no reason. Be on the lookout for radical mood changes—they might be thyroid related.

Development of the thyroid begins around the seventeenth day after conception. When the fetus reaches three months gestation, it begins to make its first thyroid hormone. During pregnancy, it also receives thyroid hormone from the mother. Even at these early stages, thyroid hormone is needed for the fetus's development of the brain and nervous system.

The thyroid gland is part of the body's endocrine system, a collection of glands that produce the hormones that regulate your growth, metabolism, and sexual development and function. Hormones— coming from a Greek word meaning "to excite" or "to spur on"—are chemical messengers that act on cells to cause chemical reactions. Once released by specific glands, they travel in the bloodstream to the targeted organ, where they spur the organ to action. Other parts of the endocrine system include the:

- Adrenal glands, which are located above the kidney, and affect metabolism, the body's stress response, and salt regulation.
- Hypothalamus, a part of the brain that regulates the pituitary gland as well as involuntary bodily functions, sleep, appetite, and hormones.

- Ovaries and testicles, which are located in the sex organs, and produce sex hormones involved in influencing female and male sexual characteristics. They regulate the menstrual cycle in women and sperm production in men.
- Pancreas, which is located below your stomach, and secretes insulin, a hormone that regulates the body's use of glucose.
- Parathyroid glands, which are located near the thyroid, and regulate calcium levels in the blood.
- Pineal gland, which is in the back of the brain, and produces melatonin, a hormone that is involved in sleep-wake cycles.
- Pituitary gland, which is located near the base of the brain, and produces numerous hormones that affect the other endocrine glands, including the thyroid.
- Thymus gland, which is located at the top of the chest, and is involved in the body's immune function.

Each one of these glands plays a vital role in keeping you healthy, and the thyroid is no exception. But the thyroid doesn't work alone. It requires help from other body parts and elements in your diet to perform the critical task of regulating metabolism and promoting healthy growth.

How the Thyroid Works

Thyroid function involves a complex interplay of several organs, various hormones, and the right nutrients. In fact, thyroid function is directly affected by two other major organs—the hypothalamus and the pituitary gland. Together, the three organs form what is sometimes called the hypothalamic-pituitary-thyroid axis, or HPT axis. The way they operate provides a glimpse of your body's highly regulated system of checks and balances.

The hypothalamus is a region of the brain that acts as an internal regulation system. It controls certain metabolic processes and autonomic activities, such as breathing, swallowing, and blinking.

The hypothalamus also links the nervous system to the endocrine system through its production of neurohormones. Of particular importance to the thyroid gland is a neurohormone called thyrotropin-releasing hormone (TRH), also called TSH-releasing hormone. TRH levels are too low to be measured in the blood and so are never used to diagnose thyroid disease.

But when thyroid hormone levels are low, TRH stimulates the pituitary gland to produce thyroid-stimulating hormone (TSH). TSH, in turn, acts on the thyroid gland to produce thyroid hormone.

But the pituitary gland doesn't sit back after the thyroid hormone is released. It continues to monitor and assess the amount of hormone in the blood. If thyroid hormone drops too low, it releases more TSH to spur on greater production of thyroid hormone. If the amount of thyroid hormone goes too high, then the pituitary gland stops releasing TSH.

TSH levels can sometimes change even when your thyroid hormones are in the normal range. But usually, when the levels of thyroid hormone are just right, the pituitary maintains its production of TSH. That's why the measure of TSH is considered the most telling of your thyroid hormone levels.

Together, the hypothalamus and the pituitary and thyroid glands work together with help from other parts of the brain to ensure that your body cells work at the proper speed. In a healthy person, this well-orchestrated feedback loop keeps your body cells functioning the way they should, much in the same way that a thermostat ensures that your house stays at a stable temperature. Even the slightest increase or decrease, however, can alter the activity in your cells. That's when disease sets in.

The Role of Iodine

These days, we hear a lot about the benefits of eating a low-sodium diet as a way to reduce hypertension. Although too much salt is undoubtedly bad for people with high blood pressure, adequate amounts of iodized salt are critical to the healthy functioning of your thyroid gland.

Iodine is a trace mineral that occurs naturally in the sea. Seafood and plants grown near saltwater, such as kelp, are natural sources of iodine. You can also find iodine in eggs and dairy products that come from chicken and cattle that have been given iodine-fortified feed. According to the American Dietetic Association, you need 150 micrograms (mcgs) of iodine a day, which is found in a half teaspoon of iodized salt. Pregnant women require 220 mcgs, and breast feeding moms need 290 mcgs.

L. Essential

People in the United States consume approximately 200 to 700 micrograms of iodine in their diets every day, according to the Thyroid Foundation of America. On the Japanese island of Hokkaido, where people consume large amounts of a seaweed called kombu, the daily iodine intake is about 200,000 micrograms. Oddly enough, people on Hokkaido don't have many thyroid problems, suggesting that normal, healthy people may naturally regulate how much iodine enters the thyroid.

These days, the primary source of iodine in North America is iodized salt. Without enough iodine in the diet, you are at risk of developing goiter, an enlarged thyroid gland. Thanks to the introduction of iodized salt in North America, goiter caused by iodine deficiency has practically been eliminated.

But in countries where iodized salt is not the norm, many people continue to suffer from iodine deficiency. In fact, iodine deficiency is the most common cause of thyroid disease worldwide. Iodine deficiency leads to goiter, and in severe cases, cretinism, severe mental retardation in infants due to iodine deficiency. Some of the areas that suffer from iodine deficiency include mountainous regions of Mexico and Central America; parts of Africa, including Ethiopia and Nigeria; parts of Asia, including India, Nepal, and China; and parts of Europe, including Italy and Switzerland.

Why is iodine so important to the thyroid? Simply put, the thyroid gland requires iodine for the production of thyroid hormones. In fact, the cells in your thyroid gland are the only ones in your body that are capable of absorbing iodine. Without it, your thyroid is totally incapable of producing the thyroid hormone that your body needs. In addition, iodine plays a significant role in the diagnosis and treatment of thyroid disease.

Once the iodine is in your body, it travels to the stomach, where it is converted to iodide. It is then transported to the thyroid gland in the blood.

Thyroid Hormone

The thyroid gland is composed of follicles, round sacs that are clustered together like tiny bubbles. The follicle consists of a gelatinous material called colloid in the center and is lined with follicular cells on the outside. These follicular cells produce thyroid hormone by absorbing iodine from the diet and combining it with thyroglobulin, a thyroid protein produced in the thyroid.

Inside each of these thyroid follicles, iodine hooks up with the thyroglobulin and mixes with an amino acid called tyrosine on the thyroglobulin to produce two forms of thyroid hormone, triiodothyronine (T3) and thyroxine (T4). The thyroid hormone is then stored in the colloid. When levels of thyroid hormone dip, the pituitary gland releases more TSH, which arrives at the thyroid follicles and attaches to TSH receptors on the cells. In the presence of TSH, T4 and T3 are cleaved off the thyroglobulin. The T4 and T3 go from the colloid back to the follicular cells and are then released into the bloodstream.

The numbers on these two forms of thyroid hormone reflect the number of iodine molecules in each molecule of thyroid hormone. In healthy people, 80 percent of the thyroid hormone you produce is T4, the less powerful form of thyroid hormone. The remaining 20 percent is T3, the more potent and active form of thyroid hormone.

The bulk of the T3 your body needs is produced by the conversion of T4 into T3. Your body cells do this conversion by removing one of the iodine molecules on T4, with help from enzymes known as deiodinases. There are three different types of these enzymes, each in different tissues. The deiodinase enzymes also convert T4 to reverse T3 (rT3), which is an inactive form of T3. The conversion of T4 into T3 takes place in organs such as the liver, kidneys, and muscles. The scientific name for the conversion process is called monodeiodination.

Fact

Follicular cells of the thyroid gland change shape depending on their activity. The cells are rectangular when the thyroid gland is active and square when it is inactive.

Once inside the bloodstream, most of the T3 and T4 hormones attach themselves to blood proteins produced by the liver, which are called thyroxine-binding globulin (TBG); thyroxine-binding prealbumin, also called transthyretin; and albumin. Only minute amounts of thyroid hormone—0.04 percent of T4 and 0.4 percent of T3—circulate in the blood as the free and active portions. The active form of thyroid hormone then travels throughout the body via the blood and binds to thyroid hormone receptors on different tissues. There are two types of thyroid receptors, TR alpha and TR beta, which have different activities.

Every single cell in your body relies on thyroid hormone to do its job. That's because thyroid hormone determines how quickly your body uses oxygen and calories from food to produce the energy cells need to do their jobs. Thyroid hormone begins doing its work at conception and continues until death.

Fact

T3 has a shorter half-life than T4, which means T4 remains in the body a lot longer than T3. Animals such as pigs have a higher amount of T3 than humans do and are used as a source for the production of natural hormone used in treatment.

Thyroid hormone has numerous and critical functions in the body, including the regulation of the speed at which individual cells function, or BMR. Here are some other ways that thyroid hormone works in your body.

- It ensures the proper growth and development of children.
- It aids in proper muscle functioning.
- It ensures that the heart pumps effectively and efficiently.
- It ensures that the gastrointestinal (GI) system is able to digest and excrete food properly.
- It strengthens hair, skin, and nails.
- It helps with the development of the brain.
- It aids in the growth of strong bones.
- It ensures proper development of the body's organs.

As you can see, thyroid hormone is a pivotal player in the proper functioning and well-being of your body. Even the slightest increase or decrease in hormone levels can affect your health.

But T4 and T3 aren't the only hormones produced by the thyroid gland. Tucked between the follicular cells are other cells, known as parafollicular cells, also called chief cells or C cells. The parafollicular cells produce calcitonin, a hormone important to bone health.

Calcitonin inhibits the removal of bone by osteoclasts, a type of cell involved in the constant breakdown of bone. These cells also produce small amounts of somatostatin, which inhibits the release of several hormones, including TSH, growth hormone, and insulin.

You may know calcitonin as a drug, not just a hormone. In postmenopausal women who have osteoporosis, calcitonin may be prescribed as a medication, under brand names such as Miacalcin and Calcimar. It works just like the natural hormone by slowing the breakdown of bone. Calcitonin is also found in salmon.

What Are the Parathyroid Glands?

Although this book is dedicated to diseases of the thyroid gland, it's important to know a little bit about the parathyroid glands. Parathyroid glands are four tiny glands—some people may have more or fewer—located behind the thyroid gland. Unlike the thyroid gland, which is made up of follicles, the parathyroid glands are composed of distinct, densely packed cells. These glands produce parathyroid hormone (PTH), which regulates the metabolism of calcium and phosphorous. They also play a role in maintaining healthy bones.

When blood-calcium levels drop below a certain point, calcium-sensing receptors in the parathyroid gland respond by releasing PTH into the blood. PTH then stimulates osteoclasts to break down bone and release calcium into the blood. By keeping the calcium levels in our body within a narrow range, our nervous and muscular systems are able to function properly.

The parathyroid glands, however, are separate and distinct from the thyroid gland. One can be healthy while the other is diseased. But the health of the parathyroid glands can be affected during thyroid surgery, which is why it's critical that the surgeon not harm the parathyroid glands during a thyroidectomy, removal of the thyroid gland.

Do a Self-Check

Thyroid disease doesn't always have signs or symptoms. When it does, the symptoms may be easily dismissed as symptoms of other conditions or lifestyle issues. Those who have symptoms directly related to their thyroid may notice a lump in their throat, hoarseness in their voice, or a pain in the neck.

In any case, one of the best ways to assess your thyroid health is to do a thyroid neck check. Because thyroid disease is so prevalent, many experts recommend performing an annual neck check on yourself—the same way women are advised to do monthly breast exams and all people are told to examine their skin. Keep in mind, however, that a self-check does not compensate for a visit to your doctor. According to the American Association of Clinical Endocrinologists (AACE), here's how to do a neck check:

1. Get a glass of water and a hand-held mirror.
2. With the mirror in your hand, study the area of your neck just below the Adam's apple and immediately above the collarbone. That is the location of your thyroid gland.
3. While focusing on this area, tip your head back.
4. Take a drink of water and swallow.
5. As you do, look at your neck. Be on the lookout for bulges or protrusions in this area when you swallow. Be careful not to confuse the Adam's apple with the thyroid gland, which is closer to the collarbone.
6. Repeat this process a few times if you suspect anything.
7. If you do see any bulges or protrusions, you should see your physician.

Many things can go wrong with the thyroid, and there are myriad tests and treatments for many types of problems. Making sense of all of them can sometimes be overwhelming. If you're not feeling well, you may already be overwhelmed and fearful about your health. You may be worried that what you have is potentially fatal. But keep in mind that knowledge is power and that information about your health is critical. It just shouldn't compound your stress.

The goal is for you to learn as much as possible about your thyroid and your particular thyroid condition. The more you know, the more quickly you'll get a diagnosis and treatment. It will also enable you to speak intelligently with your doctors and to become a partner in your ongoing care.

CHAPTER 2

The Unhealthy Thyroid

When the thyroid is well, you won't give it a second thought. But when the humble gland is diseased, your entire existence can be affected. You may gain or lose weight, feel hot or cold, and notice changes in your energy levels. In this chapter, we'll give you an overview of what happens when the thyroid isn't functioning properly.

When the Thyroid Gets Sick

Life is humming along smoothly, but one day you notice that your skin is drier than usual. Or maybe you start to feel more fatigued than normal. Or perhaps you feel anxious, uneasy, and irritable.

While it's easy to chalk up these symptoms to the weather, advancing age, or too much stress, they are also the symptoms of a thyroid problem. Too much thyroid hormone, and your body speeds up. That's hyperthyroidism. Too little thyroid hormone, and it slows down. That's called hypothyroidism.

Many things can go wrong with the thyroid. An autoimmune problem, in which the body is attacking its own healthy tissues, may trigger Hashimoto's thyroiditis and cause hypothyroidism. Or it may cause Graves' disease, which will bring on hyperthyroidism. You may also develop nodules (lumps), goiters (enlargement), or cancer. Your thyroid may also be affected by pregnancy and advancing age.

📋 Fact

When it comes to autoimmune diseases, which include lupus, type 1 diabetes, and Addison's disease, the odds are stacked against women. In fact, about 75 percent of all autoimmune diseases occur in women, leaving experts to speculate that hormones play a role. Autoimmune diseases are also among the most poorly understood and recognized forms of disease, says the American Autoimmune Related Diseases Association.

Each disease creates its own signs and symptoms, some more disturbing and noticeable than others. The good news is, most problems with the thyroid are easily treated. Left untreated, however, thyroid disease can cause some serious complications, even death.

Factors That Increase Risk

Anyone can develop thyroid disease, but certain factors make you more likely to develop a thyroid problem than the person who doesn't have that risk. At the same time, having these risk factors doesn't guarantee that you'll have a thyroid problem. Following are some of the main risk factors that can affect thyroid health.

Gender and Age

No doubt, being a woman makes you more vulnerable to thyroid disease. In fact, according to the American Association of Clinical Endocrinologists, one in eight women between the ages of thirty-five and sixty-five has thyroid disease, most cases hypothyroidism. And as you age, the risk gets even higher: 20 percent of all women over sixty-five have thyroid problems.

Being female is also the biggest risk factor for Graves' disease, which afflicts women eight times more often than men. But Graves' is not necessarily a condition of advancing age. Rather, most people develop Graves' disease between ages twenty and forty.

Personal and Family Health History

If you've ever had a problem with your thyroid in the past, your risk for thyroid disease now is higher than normal. For instance, even a brief thyroid problem after pregnancy makes you more vulnerable.

You are also at greater risk for an autoimmune thyroid disease if you have an autoimmune condition such as rheumatoid arthritis, scleroderma, lupus, or psoriasis. Two forms of thyroid disease, Hashimoto's disease and Graves' disease, are also autoimmune illnesses. A discussion of other diseases that might raise your risk for thyroid disorders appears later in this chapter.

The same risk applies to your family members. If a first-degree relative has had or has thyroid disease, then you are more likely to have a thyroid problem. For instance, if your mother had a bout of postpartum thyroid disease after delivery years ago, your risk is slightly higher than someone whose mom didn't have the condition.

But remember, having a personal or family history of thyroid disease or autoimmune disease doesn't mean you will necessarily get thyroid disease. It simply means that your chances of doing so are slightly higher than those of a person who doesn't have that history.

Cigarette Smoking

It's safe to say that everyone knows about the toll that cigarettes have on the health of our lungs and hearts. But smoking cigarettes also causes serious problems for the thyroid. In fact, one recent study identified cigarette smoking as a predictor of Graves' disease.

For these reasons—among so many others—people with a personal or family history of thyroid disease or autoimmune illnesses are generally advised not to smoke. And if you find out you do have thyroid disease, do everything you can to quit.

Alert

> Giving up the cigarette habit is difficult, to say the least. And 21 per-
> cent of the U.S. population still lights up despite efforts to nix the
> habit. The Centers for Disease Control and Prevention offers a listing
> of useful Internet resources that can help you quit. For information,
> check out: *www.cdc.gov/tobacco/how2quit.htm.*

Hormonal Upheaval

Many women will develop thyroid disease during periods of tremendous hormonal shifts, especially during or after pregnancy and
just before or during menopause. Approximately 10 percent of all
women will develop some form of thyroid disease after pregnancy.
In fact, some women will develop a condition called postpartum thyroiditis, an inflammation of the thyroid gland that usually lasts just
six to nine months, then disappears on its own. It is often the reason
for postpartum depression.

Thyroid disease also occurs around the time of menopause. But
because the timing of thyroid disease often coincides with these hormonal shifts, many women go undiagnosed. Patients and physicians
alike often assume that their symptoms are related to their reproductive hormones, not their thyroid.

Exposure to Radiation

Say the word *Chernobyl*, and most people will recall the 1986
nuclear tragedy in Ukraine. One of the subsequent results of that
nuclear disaster has been a higher incidence of thyroid disease in
the region, including thyroid cancer in children. Studies suggest that
exposing the thyroid gland to significant radiation can raise your
risk for thyroid disease, including thyroid cancer. However, routine
X-rays—as long as you're not pregnant—are unlikely to increase the
odds for developing thyroid disease.

What is of concern is radiation done to the head, neck, and throat, such as that used to treat cancers in those parts of the body. For instance, people with Hodgkin's disease who are treated with radiation are at greater risk for thyroid disease. In addition, studies have found that women who undergo multiple X-rays during pregnancy were more likely to give birth to low-weight babies, an effect that the researchers attributed to the probable effect the X-rays had on the thyroid.

Having a Medical Condition

The presence of certain illnesses may actually suggest a thyroid problem. For example, fibromyalgia, a condition characterized by widespread pain and fatigue, and chronic fatigue immune deficiency syndrome (CFIDS), a similar condition marked by persistent and debilitating fatigue, may be due to an undiagnosed thyroid problem and suggest that you need to see an endocrinologist. The same is true if you have an endocrine disorder such as diabetes.

Thyroid problems are also more common in women who have endometriosis, in which the tissue lining of the uterus grows outside the uterus, and in those who have polycystic ovarian syndrome (PCOS), a condition characterized by irregular periods, excess facial and body hair, infertility, and tiny cysts around the ovaries. In addition, thyroid disease is more prevalent in people who have celiac disease, an intolerance of gluten.

The most apparent link between thyroid disease and other conditions occurs in autoimmune problems: people who already have an autoimmune disease, such as lupus, rheumatoid arthritis, or scleroderma, are at increased risk for thyroid disease.

Other Risk Factors

Many people are convinced that other factors are at play in the development of thyroid disease. Some suggest it might be linked to stress. Others suggest it might be the result of a viral or bacterial infection, or the result of physical trauma to the thyroid gland. Even premature graying and being left-handed have been cited as risk factors for thyroid disease.

Fact

Our modern understanding of the thyroid is relatively recent. In fact, Theodor Kocher, a Swiss surgeon, was the first doctor to remove the thyroid gland for the treatment of goiter. It was Kocher who realized the profound impact of the thyroid on growth and body functions. In 1909, he received a Nobel Prize in medicine for his work on the thyroid gland.

No single risk factor has been identified as a definite cause for thyroid disease. All we know is that you are more likely to develop thyroid problems if you have one or more of these risk factors.

Things That Can Go Wrong

When it's healthy, the thyroid gland quietly performs its tasks like an unsung hero, a quiet but instrumental cog in the marvelous machine known as the human body. But when it gets diseased, the problems can become annoying at best, and life-threatening at worst.

Thyroid disease is actually several medical conditions, each with its own set of signs and symptoms. The following is an overview of these different conditions.

Hypothyroidism

Inexplicable weight gain. Fatigue. Memory loss. In people whose thyroid gland doesn't produce enough thyroid hormone, the result is a slowing down of all bodily functions, causing a condition called hypothyroidism.

Hypothyroidism is the most common form of thyroid disease. Although it can be temporary in some cases, most often it is a permanent medical condition that requires lifelong medication and vigilance. People who have it may notice that they feel sluggish, depressed, and unable to concentrate. But in its milder forms, they may notice nothing at all. Some people, like Susan, have no symptoms at all. In fact, it was family history that inspired Susan to have her thyroid checked:

> When Susan told her nurse practitioner that her sister had been diagnosed with Hashimoto's, the nurse practitioner suggested she get screened, even though she had no symptoms. Sure enough, they found that Susan had it, too. She was immediately put on thyroid hormone replacement and notices she has more energy.

Many factors can cause an underactive thyroid, but the most common one is an autoimmune disease called Hashimoto's thyroiditis (or disease). In an autoimmune disease, the body's immune system mistakenly treats healthy tissue as a foreign invader, and attacks its own body cells. But hypothyroidism can also be caused by inflammation, radioactive iodine treatments for hyperthyroidism, removal of the thyroid gland—possibly as a result of cancer—certain medications, and problems with the pituitary gland.

Essential

Children who have Down's syndrome are more likely to develop hypothyroidism. The two conditions, as they appear in children, share similar features. Hypothyroidism, if severe, like Down's syndrome, can involve mental retardation and slow growth. Treating the hypothyroidism is still important, however, and can improve a child's growth and functioning.

Some women develop hypothyroidism during or after pregnancy, and some children are born with a deficiency in hormone production or thyroid tissue. In some cases, the cause of the hypothyroidism may remain a mystery.

Mild Hypothyroidism

Some cases of hypothyroidism are less clear-cut. TSH levels may be normal or near normal, but you may still be experiencing all the symptoms of hypothyroidism. Some doctors may be uncertain about whether to treat you. This condition is known as mild, or subclinical, hypothyroidism.

Doctors who consider TSH levels only in making a diagnosis may say you do not have hypothyroidism at all. But those who consider the symptoms you're experiencing as well as your TSH levels may be more inclined to say you are hypothyroid and give you thyroid hormone replacement.

In any case, people who have mild hypothyroidism may have the same symptoms as those with hypothyroidism—fatigue, weight gain, and depression. Some experts believe that treating mild hypothyroidism can prevent a patient from developing full-blown hypothyroidism.

Hyperthyroidism

Unexplained weight loss. Nervousness. A fast heartbeat. In people whose thyroid glands are producing too much thyroid hormone, the body speeds up, and the result is a less well-known thyroid condition called hyperthyroidism.

Hyperthyroidism afflicts about 1 percent of the U.S. population, and affects women five to ten times more often than men. People who have it are jittery, anxious, and have trouble catching their breath. They may be plagued by insomnia and notice that their eyes bulge. In milder forms, hyperthyroidism may produce no symptoms at all.

Many cases of hyperthyroidism are caused by Graves' disease, an autoimmune condition that causes enlargement of the thyroid gland. But it may also be the result of the growth of several nodules in the thyroid, a single nodule, inflammation and enlargement of the thyroid gland (called thyroiditis), or the overingestion of iodine. Some people who are taking thyroid medication for hypothyroidism may become hyperthyroid too, if they take too much medication. In some women, hyperthyroidism may develop after pregnancy.

Goiters

Before the introduction of iodized salt in the 1920s, the United States was plagued with goiter, which is an enlargement of the thyroid gland. Goiters may be the result of too much or too little thyroid hormone, and they are not cancerous. Some patients with a goiter may have hypo- or hyperthyroidism. Others may have normal thyroid tests and still have a goiter.

But goiters can develop if you have either hypothyroidism or hyperthyroidism. In people with underactive thyroids, inadequate amounts of thyroid hormone cause TSH levels to go up, spurring the development of a goiter. Goiters that result from hypothyroidism in the United States are most often caused by Hashimoto's disease. Goiters may also be the result of an overactive thyroid brought on by Graves' disease, which causes the gland to swell and enlarge. Elsewhere in the world, where iodine deficiencies are more common, the goiter may be caused by inadequate intake of iodine.

Fact

The Great Lakes region, the Midwest, and the mountainous regions of the interior United States were once called the "goiter belt," areas of the country where goiter was prevalent because of iodine deficiency. That problem was remedied with the introduction of iodized salt in the 1920s.

Goiters also occur when you have other thyroid problems. In some people, a goiter may be the result of a single nodule, or multiple nodules, a condition called multinodular goiter. You may also develop a goiter as the result of inflammation of the thyroid gland.

Some women may develop a goiter during pregnancy as the result of a hormone called human chorionic gonadotropin (HCG).

Thyroid Nodules

Simply put, a nodule is a lump. The vast majority of thyroid nodules are small, benign (noncancerous), and harmless. They may occur as a single nodule or as a clump.

Most thyroid nodules are stealth invaders. You may not even notice you have a nodule until your doctor feels one in your throat during a routine physical. But if the nodule gets bigger, you may see it on your throat as a lump in the lower front of your neck. Women may see it when they're applying makeup. Men may notice it while they're shaving or if their shirt collars begin to feel uncomfortably snug.

Large nodules may actually press against your windpipe or your esophagus, making it difficult for you to breathe or swallow. They may even cause hoarseness in your voice.

L. Essential

Even a benign nodule may sometimes warrant surgical removal. If the nodule becomes so big that it interferes with breathing and swallowing, surgery can remove the obstruction and alleviate the pressure. You may also consider removing it if the nodule becomes large and unsightly.

Although most nodules are benign, in some cases, the nodule may be cancerous. A single nodule in an otherwise healthy gland, a nodule that is hard to the touch, or one that doesn't shrink after thyroid hormone treatments are all signs that your nodule may be cancerous. Nodules accompanied by enlargement of the lymph nodes in the neck may also indicate cancer. The bottom line is this: All nodules warrant medical attention and evaluation to pin down the exact cause and type of nodule.

Thyroid Cancer

There are four distinct types of thyroid cancer: papillary, follicular, medullary, and anaplastic. Each form develops in different cells of the thyroid gland and is distinct from the others. Although having cancer can be frightening to anyone, most cases of thyroid cancer are readily treated with surgery. And though having thyroid cancer means you'll need regular monitoring to detect any recurrence, most patients go on to live normal, productive lives.

Alert

Vigilance is everything when it comes to thyroid cancer, which has a recurrence rate of about 30 percent. Sometimes, the cancer returns decades after the initial diagnosis. Monitor your thyroid health regularly with routine visits to the doctor, blood tests, physical exams, and imaging techniques. Make these doctor visits a top priority.

The incidence of thyroid cancer has increased in recent years. And like most other thyroid problems, the condition is more common in women than men. Your risk also goes up if you were exposed to radiation as a child or if you have a family history of thyroid cancer.

Euthyroid Sick Syndrome

You're in the hospital for heart problems when the doctor announces your thyroid is off-kilter, too. These abnormal findings in the absence of thyroid disease is what experts call euthyroid sick syndrome. People with this condition have not had thyroid problems in the past but are now experiencing abnormalities because of another medical problem.

Euthyroid sick syndrome—sometimes called sick euthyroid—can occur with many illnesses, including cardiovascular disease, pulmonary disease, and renal problems. It may also occur with gastrointestinal disease, inflammatory conditions, and sepsis. Some people have it after surgery, trauma, or burns.

In most cases, levels of T3 are low, and reverse T3 is high, a condition called low T3 syndrome. It's possible that when the body is ill, reducing the amount of T3—and thereby slowing bodily functions—is the body's way of conserving its resources. But in other cases, other thyroid hormones may be involved. For instance, if the euthyroid sick syndrome is severe, both T3 and T4 levels drop. And among the sickest patients, TSH levels become abnormally low.

The good news is, euthyroid sick syndrome is usually a temporary problem. As patients recover from their illness, their TSH levels may rise to hypothyroid levels until thyroid hormone levels stabilize. Eventually, all thyroid hormones become normal again.

Most experts agree that euthyroid sick syndrome is not hypothyroidism in spite of the drop in hormone levels. But many doctors are now finding that treatment with T3 has benefits. For instance, those who are suffering from heart failure may experience an improvement in their heart's pumping capacity after being treated with T3, even though they technically do not have a thyroid disorder. As a result, doctors these days are increasingly inclined to treat euthyroid sick syndrome.

A Great Imitator

Now that you know something about all the thyroid does for your health, you may be baffled why anyone would overlook a thyroid problem. After all, wouldn't you notice if you were putting on weight without overeating? Or if your skin were drying out or you felt more sluggish than usual?

In reality, the thyroid is often overlooked, ignored, or dismissed as the source of your suffering and symptoms. That's because the symptoms of thyroid disease mimic those of other conditions as well as common lifestyle issues. You're gaining weight because you're getting older. Your skin is dry because it's winter, and the heat is on. You're sluggish because you're working long hours and raising kids. Many other factors in your life can make it easy for you to dismiss your symptoms as anything more than minor inconveniences.

At the same time, you may suspect your thyroid when, in reality, your symptoms are actually the result of another medical condition. Many conditions produce symptoms that resemble those that occur in thyroid disease. (*Note:* As you go over this list, you'll notice that many of these conditions are the same ones that may elevate your risk for thyroid disease.) Depending on the symptoms you have and the type of thyroid disease, these imitators might include:

- Chronic fatigue immune deficiency syndrome
- Fibromyalgia
- Menopause
- Depression
- Anxiety and panic attacks
- Arthritis
- Sleep apnea
- Diabetes and insulin resistance
- Irritable bowel syndrome

If you notice that your neck looks larger than usual or recall that your mother once had thyroid problems, you may want to reconsider your thyroid as the source of your health problems. But remember, thyroid disease is not always apparent in your neck. Only a blood test can help determine whether your thyroid is the culprit.

Thyroid Disease and the Rest of Your Body

As you know, the thyroid gland affects virtually every aspect of your well-being. So it should be no surprise that a sick thyroid can wreak havoc on many aspects of your health and put you at risk for other health problems. The ways in which thyroid disease can affect you are many and varied. Below is a partial list of some of the potentially major problems you might experience. Fortunately, most of these problems are resolved with prompt and proper treatment.

Eye Disease

The eyes are sensitive to the effects of thyroid hormone. Nowhere is that more apparent than in people who have hyperthyroidism. Almost everyone who has hyperthyroidism will develop a stare in which the eyes appear to have a wide-eyed, startled appearance.

People who have Graves' disease often develop a separate condition called thyroid eye disease, or infiltrative ophthalmology. A distinct bulging of the eyeball occurs as a result of swelling in the muscles around the eyes, which pushes the eyeball forward. Some people may have difficulty closing their eyes completely, which leads to redness and irritation of the eyeball.

In more severe cases, the eyes may not move in sync, and you may experience double vision. You may also notice that your eyes are more sensitive to light, and that they frequently feel gritty, dry, and irritated.

Cholesterol Levels

In people who have hypothyroidism, cholesterol levels may become elevated. In particular, an underactive thyroid raises levels of low-density lipoprotein, or LDL, the "bad" cholesterol that promotes heart disease.

Unless you have a blood test, you won't know that you have high cholesterol or that your LDL levels have gone up. But it's important to keep tabs on your cholesterol if you do have hypothyroidism. Cholesterol is the waxy fatlike substance that clogs arteries, and too much of it can lead to heart disease or even a heart attack.

Likewise, if blood tests show that you have high cholesterol, ask for a thyroid test as a follow-up. An underactive thyroid can make it hard for your body to metabolize. In fact, the average cholesterol level for someone with hypothyroidism is 250 mg/dL, well above the 200 mg/dL recommended for good health. Treating thyroid disease can lower your cholesterol.

Depression and Anxiety

The thyroid gland has a powerful effect on mood. Many people with thyroid disease may notice that they feel depressed. Depression is a serious mood disorder that frequently involves feelings of sadness, emptiness, helplessness, and hopelessness. You may withdraw from others and lose pleasure in activities you once enjoyed.

In people who have hyperthyroidism, the depression may coexist with major mood swings. Some people may experience bouts of mania and elation interspersed with erratic bouts of crying and sadness. The erratic moods may even cause bizarre behavior.

Some people with an overactive thyroid may experience anxiety, which can make you edgy, irritable, nervous, and fearful. Others may develop a panic disorder, which causes similar symptoms, such as heart palpitations, trouble catching your breath, numbness, and sweating or chills. In fact, some people may be diagnosed with panic disorder when the problem is really an overactive thyroid.

Heart Problems

A faulty thyroid gland can take a toll on the heart as well. A recent study in the *Archives of Internal Medicine* found that people with even subclinical (mild) hypothyroidism had higher rates of heart disease. The risk for heart disease may be largely linked to higher cholesterol levels caused by even the slightest decrease in thyroid hormone levels.

Essential

Your pulse tells you how many times your heart beats in a minute. To take your pulse, place two fingers gently on the artery on the palm side of your wrist. Do not use your thumb, which has its own pulse. Count the number of beats in 30 seconds, and multiply it by two. A normal pulse is 50 to 100 beats per minute. To get your normal resting pulse, sit still for 10 minutes before taking your pulse.

In people with hyperthyroidism, the heart may beat too rapidly or erratically, causing palpitations. When the heart beats too fast and too strong for a long time, you may experience heart failure, a potentially fatal condition that causes shortness of breath, swelling, and fluid in your lungs.

In some cases, an overactive thyroid gland can lead to atrial fibrillation, an abnormal heart rhythm that raises your risk for spontaneous blood clots that could lead to a stroke. This condition is most common in people who already have a heart problem. It is quite serious and warrants attention from a cardiologist.

Weight Problems

For someone who always wanted to lose weight, an overactive thyroid might seem like a blessing at first. People with hyperthyroidism are prone to weight loss, even as their appetites surge. Sometimes, however, they may experience weight gain because they're eating so much to compensate for their body's demand for more energy. People who have hypothyroidism, on the other hand, tend to gain weight even as their appetite declines.

Other Problems

These are just a few of the more serious ways that a malfunctioning thyroid can affect your health. But thyroid disease can also affect many other aspects of your health, including your hair, skin, nails, digestive tract, and muscles. It can take a toll on your energy levels, your sleep habits, and your ability to concentrate. It can affect your fertility and make it difficult for you to get pregnant. If it goes untreated, it can eventually even affect your ability to function and perform your job.

In later chapters, you'll read about how the thyroid gland affects other parts of your body. But as you can see, the impact of the thyroid can affect your health in many ways. Again, the key to preventing problems from worsening is prompt diagnosis and treatment.

CHAPTER 3

Choosing a Thyroid Doctor

A good doctor isn't always easy to find. Finding a good thyroid doctor can be even more challenging. But a skilled physician is going to be extremely important to someone with thyroid disease, especially since many of these conditions involve lifelong management. In this chapter, you'll learn how to tell the good docs from the bad, find out where specialists play into the picture, and discover what it takes to create a strong doctor-patient relationship.

From Primary Care to Endocrinology

Chances are, the first doctor you'll see is your primary care doctor. You might go in complaining of fatigue and weight gain, or you may go in after you've noticed a bump in your neck. Alternatively, you may be on a routine physical exam when your doctor detects an abnormal lump in your thyroid. In any case, your primary care doctor is often your first stop on the way to diagnosing and treating your thyroid troubles.

Some cases of thyroid disease go no further than your primary care doctor, who may be perfectly qualified to detect the source of your thyroid problems. Some primary care doctors are suitably qualified to treat an under- or overactive thyroid. These doctors are often internists, who specialize in internal medicine; family practitioners, physicians who treat families; or general practitioners.

Some people have as their primary care doctor an osteopathic physician (DO). Osteopathic doctors are trained just like medical doctors and are able to prescribe medications and perform routine examinations. What makes DOs different from MDs is that their training emphasizes viewing the body as an integrated whole.

Ü Question

What is a thyroidologist?
It's arguable whether the term thyroidologist is real. There is no board certification to be a thyroidologist, only for endocrinologists. But doctors who call themselves thyroidologists specialize in disorders of the thyroid. Endocrinologists can treat the entire endocrine system but may specialize in one aspect of it. If your primary doctor suspects you have a more serious thyroid problem, she may feel more comfortable sending you to a specialist, usually an endocrinologist.

Meet Your Endocrinologist

Endocrinologists specialize in the treatment and care of hormone disorders, such as thyroid disease, reproductive disorders, and diabetes. For many people with thyroid disease, an endocrinologist is their primary care doctor—the first one they call when something goes wrong with a new drug or when they feel symptoms.

Becoming an endocrinologist requires rigorous medical training. After four years of medical school, an endocrinologist must spend three or four years in an internship and residency program. Beyond that, they focus exclusively on hormonal disorders for another two or three years before becoming board certified in endocrinology. Many endocrinologists are fellows of the AACE, a membership that is signified by the initials FACE. However, not all endocrinologists are knowledgeable in thyroid disease. Rather, they may specialize in diabetes, lipid disorders, or reproductive endocrinology.

Many academic endocrinologists are members of the Endocrine Society, the professional arm of the Hormone Foundation. This prestigious organization hosts yearly meetings that expose endocrinologists to the latest research. A list of members can be found on the Internet at *www.endo-society.org/apps/FindAnEndo/index.cfm*.

Certain people with thyroid disease are more apt to need the services of an endocrinologist than others. These include people who have:

- Mild hypothyroidism
- Hypothyroidism due to a pituitary disorder
- Graves' disease
- Thyroid nodules
- Thyroid cancer
- A condition that requires thyroid surgery

Others may simply prefer to see an endocrinologist if they develop thyroid disease. After all, an endocrinologist is generally more familiar with disorders involving the hormones than most other physicians are.

If you want or need to see an endocrinologist, you can probably ask your primary care doctor for a referral. But you may also want to ask friends, family members, and other people with thyroid disease for referrals. You can also look for an endocrinologist on the Internet or in chat rooms about thyroid disease. Many doctors now have their own Web site and frequently communicate with patients by e-mail.

Ideally, you'll find a good doctor you genuinely like, since thyroid problems can last a lifetime and will require lifelong maintenance.

What Makes a Good Endocrinologist?

Not all doctors are created equal. Some may be technically competent but lack the people skills that prompt patients to open up about embarrassing but important symptoms. Others may be great communicators but neglect to stay on top of the latest developments in endocrine research. When it comes to finding the best endocrinologist to treat your thyroid disease, you want one who is both skilled and com-passionate, namely, someone you can trust.

L. Essential

Love your doctor? Nominate him on Mary J. Shomon's About .com site, *http://thyroid.about.com* (go to the Top Thyroid Doctors Directory). The site allows you to click on a state and read what other patients have to say about their doctors. It also gives the top docs' addresses, phone numbers, and e-mail addresses.

It isn't always easy to find someone who meets those high stan-dards. Some doctors treat their patients according to the results of their lab tests, while others are more inclined to consider a patient's symptoms only. Ideally, you will find a doctor who considers both factors in making a diagnosis and deciding on treatment.

Doing some research before you start seeing a doctor can help you find a good physician. After all, having a chronic condition means you'll be seeing a lot more of the health-care profession. It will also mean working more closely with your doctors on matters important to your well-being.

So even if the doctor comes to you from your mother, you may find him unsuitable in ways that don't bother your mom.

Some good questions to ask his staff include:

- Does the physician specialize in the treatment of thyroid disease?
- Does he already have many patients with thyroid disease? Does he have a long waiting list?
- What kinds of alliances does the physician have with other health-care professionals? Is she plugged in to a network of other medical professionals or affiliated with a good hospital?

- Are there other people in her practice who can assist in your care?
- What kind of health insurance does the doctor accept?
- Would it upset him if you sought a second opinion?
- What does he think of alternative therapies?
- How convenient is the office to your home or workplace?

On your first few encounters, take note of the doctor's communication skills. Does he speak clearly, in words you understand, and answer your questions? Does he make you feel comfortable in his presence? Does he call back when you need assistance or information?

Also, take note of the office support staff. Schedulers, nurses, and assistants who are courteous and respectful can make a big difference in how well you do with your doctor. They can also affect how likely you are to see your doctor when you really need him.

Keep in mind, too, that the best doctor may not be the one who is closest to you. In more complicated cases, you may need to travel quite a distance to find the best doctor.

What to Expect from a Good Doctor

We all have expectations of the people we hire. Doctors should be no different. When you choose a doctor to treat you for thyroid disease, you should look for someone who first and foremost believes that your symptoms are real. The doctor should also have confidence in finding relief for your symptoms. He should be well versed in all facets of thyroid disease and be on top of the research that's going on. A doctor who is actually involved in research and attends meetings on thyroid disease, for instance, demonstrates a commitment to knowing as much as possible.

She should also be an effective communicator who can speak to you in comprehensible terms without using complex medical terminology. At the same time, she needs to be a good listener, even when you're challenging her or telling her you'd like a second opinion. She should always invite you to ask questions and offer ideas.

✎ Alert

No patient should ever tolerate a doctor who is rude, insensitive, and dismissive of your complaints and concerns. You also shouldn't tolerate a doctor who doesn't speak to you in comprehensible terms, or who routinely passes you off to his staff. Your doctor should also have a plan to diagnose and treat you. Remember, you are the client, and you have the right to "fire" your doctor.

Finally, a good doctor should be open, honest, and forthcoming with information. She should be willing to provide you with any report or information you want, even when the news is bad.

Specialists You Might Need

In some people, thyroid disease requires more than just an endocrinologist or your primary care doctor. For instance, if you have Graves' disease and develop eye problems, you may need an ophthalmologist. If you have thyroid cancer, you may need a surgeon to remove your thyroid. If your thyroid problems begin to affect your emotional state, you may require the services of a psychiatrist. And almost everyone with thyroid disease needs a good pharmacist who can spot potential drug interactions.

Finding these specialists often begins with your primary care doctor. If you're lucky, you'll get a good referral, and that's good enough. But if you don't like the specialist your doctor recommends, check around with friends and family again, or do your own research on the Internet. You can also go back to your primary doctor for another recommendation. Here are some of the key players who might wind up on your medical team.

Doctor in Nuclear Medicine

The use of radioactive iodine in the treatment of thyroid disorders has been around since the 1940s. But even though the treatment is nothing new, it does require a doctor who is skilled in the use of nuclear medicine and who works in a facility in compliance with the laws of your state.

According to the Society of Nuclear Medicine, doctors who administer radioactive iodine (RAI) should be board certified in nuclear medicine, radiology, or radiation oncology, "or be able to document equivalent training, competency, and experience in the safe use and administration of I-131," which is iodine-131, the isotope most commonly used.

Doctors who pursue a career in nuclear medicine train for at least three years after graduating from medical school. They must go through a year of preparatory training in a program approved by the Accreditation Council for Graduate Medical Education (ACGME) and then two or more years of a nuclear medicine residency in a program accredited by the ACGME. They also receive training in clinical nuclear medicine and in other health sciences. Generally, it is your endocrinologist who refers you to a doctor who specializes in nuclear medicine.

Thyroid Surgeon

Several kinds of doctors are able to do surgical procedures on the thyroid. General surgeons; head and neck surgeons; and ear, nose, and throat surgeons are all potentially capable of doing thyroid surgery. But the most important criterion for your choice of a surgeon is the surgeon's experience. The amount of experience the surgeon has is inversely related to the complications rate—that means the more experienced the surgeon, the less likely you'll suffer complications.

Judging a surgeon's experience involves asking some simple questions ahead of time. In addition to those above that you might ask a doctor, good questions for a surgeon include:

- **How many thyroid surgeries do you do in a year?** Ideally, the surgeon should do twenty to twenty-five surgeries. Some people—including the New York Thyroid Center—recommend looking for surgeons who do fifty a year.

- **How many thyroid surgeries have you done in your career?** Again, the more surgeries a surgeon has done, the better skilled he is. Someone who has done 500 or more procedures is generally considered experienced, according to the New York Thyroid Center.
- **What kind of training did you have?** A skilled surgeon will discuss any specialty training he might have had in endocrine surgery—and specifically thyroid surgery.
- **Are you involved in research in thyroid disease?** Involvement in any type of thyroid research is a good indicator that the surgeon is interested in learning as much as possible about the thyroid.

Ophthalmologist

In people who have Graves' disease, the eyes may be affected. That's when you might need the help of an ophthalmologist, a medical doctor who treats the eyes. Unlike an optometrist, an ophthalmologist can prescribe medications and do surgery.

Eye problems that result from Graves' disease are called Graves' ophthalmology. In the scheme of eye disorders, this is a relatively rare condition. For the best treatment and care, you should find an ophthalmologist who specializes in thyroid-related eye disease. These doctors are more likely to have the skills, expertise, and resources to treat your eye problems. And in the event you need surgery to correct your eye disease, you will most definitely want an ophthalmologist who specializes in thyroid-related eye disease.

Mental Health Professional

It's not unusual for serious health problems to affect your mental well-being. Many patients wind up suffering from depression or anxiety as a result of their health issues. If you are one of them, you should seek out a mental health professional. Don't be shy about getting this kind of help. Mood disorders like depression can be very serious and affect your ability to take care of yourself.

Mental health professionals can come from many backgrounds, including psychiatry, psychology, social work, and counseling. A psychiatrist is a medical doctor who, in addition to counseling and therapy, can prescribe medications. A psychologist is a mental health professional who can offer counseling and do psychotherapy but is not a medical doctor. Some people may also need a psychopharmacologist, a psychiatrist who specializes in administering medicines for difficult psychiatric problems.

Social workers are people who have at least a master's degree in social work and may provide counseling services. Some people may also seek counseling from a trusted clergy person.

Pharmacist

Before you got sick, you probably saw a pharmacist only a few times a year. But if you have a thyroid disorder, your pharmacist may become an important ally.

Pharmacists can alert you to potentially dangerous drug interactions and possible side effects from any medications you're prescribed. They can tell you whether an over-the-counter remedy or herbal supplement will interact with a prescription medication you're taking. They can also advise you on whether you should take certain drugs with food or on an empty stomach. A good relationship with a pharmacist can become vital to your health, so choose one you like, and use that person for all your prescriptions.

You're the Boss

It's easy to defer to your doctor when it comes to medical problems. After all, your doctor is the trained professional who knows the fancy five-syllable words. And in reality, he may know considerably more than you do about how your thyroid functions, the diagnostic tools you need to pinpoint the problem, and what you need to get well. On the other hand, if you've been doing your research, your knowledge may surpass your physician's.

The bottom line is this: If you don't like the way a doctor handles your care, you have the right to demand better treatment—or to go to another doctor. It's ultimately up to you whether you'll use that person's services.

Being in charge also means you have to be assertive about what you want and need. So if you've always felt uncomfortable talking to your primary care doctor or disliked the staff that made your appointments and took your phone calls, now is the time to do something and find someone new.

The key to spearheading any team—sports, corporate, or health care—is knowing what you want. In this case, you should figure out what you want from your health-care providers. Do you want someone whose office hours match your work hours? Does the office location make a difference? Do you prefer young doctors fresh out of medical school or doctors who've been in practice for several years? The answers to these questions can help you zero in on the doctors who will make up your team.

Essential

If you've just been diagnosed with a thyroid disorder, make sure you schedule a follow-up visit a few weeks after your first visit. Anticipate regular visits after that, so your doctor can check whether the medications are working. Regular visits to your doctor are now a part of your routine, and critical to your health and well-being. Some doctors will also follow up by e-mail or phone.

The Doctor-Patient Relationship

You think you've found the perfect doctor. She's got all the right credentials, a warm and friendly manner, and a nice support staff, too. She even has ideal office hours in a good location. Now, it's time to get to the business of diagnosing what's wrong and making sure that you stay healthy. Like any relationship, you want it to get off to a good start.

The First Visit

Once you've located the right doctor, you will need to make time for a thorough exam and evaluation. Make sure to set aside enough time for this appointment so you won't feel rushed, especially if you get delayed. This first visit is critical to helping your doctor make a diagnosis and determine your need for further testing and any work with specialists. Most important, it will set the tone for the future of your relationship.

Among the things you can expect at this first visit are:

- A frank and thorough discussion of your symptoms, when they began and how they're affecting you
- A detailed medical history of you and your family
- Descriptions of any changes in your health, such as changes in appetite, sleep patterns, weight loss or gain, and cognitive function
- Discussions about your lifestyle, including diet and exercise habits, and your consumption of drugs and alcohol

A thorough physical examination and open, honest dialogue are important to help your doctor rule out other health problems. So don't be hesitant to discuss all your health concerns. You may find it embarrassing that you're having more frequent bowel movements or that your libido is low, but your doctor will find it useful information toward a proper diagnosis. Remember, he's probably heard it all before.

Keep Good Records

Now that you've assembled a medical team, it's up to you to serve as its leader. That means it's up to you to keep track of what's going on with your tests, appointments, and medications.

A big part of that job is keeping well-organized medical records. Doctors see hundreds of patients a year, and it can get hard to keep track of which patient takes which medication, or when he last saw you. When it comes time to see you, he'll rely on what you tell him to help him figure out what to do next. In addition, doctors can move, so it's a good idea to start keeping those records right from the start. Good medical records should include information about the following.

Your Medications

You should always keep with you an updated list of all medications you take, including the dose of your pills and when you take them. You should also keep a separate list of medicines you have tried, including the dose used and why you stopped using it, which can help your doctors decide what to prescribe.

 Alert

If you choose to enlist an alternative health practitioner—such as a homeopath or chiropractor—use that treatment to complement your thyroid care, not replace the treatment of your primary doctor or endocrinologist. Also, be wary of any doctor who promises you quick relief, a special diet for your weight problems, or even a cure. If something sounds too good to be true, it probably is.

Any Doctor Visit

Record all your doctor visits, even dental checkups, in one place. Write down the date you went, the purpose of your visit, any symptoms you were experiencing, and any medications or therapies you were prescribed. Also record your weight and blood pressure.

Consultation Reports from Specialists

Any time you see a specialist, ask for a report of the visit. These typed narrative reports, sometimes addressed to your primary care doctor, provide comprehensive descriptions of your symptoms, what happened during the exam, and any lab findings. The specialist may also offer an analysis of the problem and a plan of action.

All Tests

Whenever your doctor orders blood work for a TSH test, an ultrasound, or an X-ray, make sure to ask for a copy, too. You might want to store this information on a spreadsheet on your computer. Over time, these reports can reveal how your health is changing. For instance, an annual increase in your blood-sugar levels may alert you to impending diabetes. If necessary, give the receptionist a self-addressed stamped envelope to ensure you get the information. Some doctors may even send the results or dictations by e-mail.

Preventive Screenings

When you have a chronic condition, it's important to keep track of all medical information, even preventive screenings that show you are healthy. Down the road, that information can establish a pattern. For instance, even if your bone-density tests are still in the normal range, they can, over time, reveal a decrease in density that may show you to be at risk for osteoporosis.

Discharge Summaries

If you're hospitalized, the attending physician will write up a summary of your visit, the procedures you underwent, the diagnosis, and your health status. If you have an outpatient procedure, ask for an operative report, which details your visit.

Be a Good Patient

It's easy for patients to gripe when their doctors are rude, arrogant, and perpetually late. But patients can be problematic, too. To get the most out of your doctor, you have to do your part in this vital relationship and be a good patient. That means you should always arrive on time and call the office to let them know when you're running late.

As the patient, it's important that you communicate openly and honestly with your doctor. Ask questions whenever you're uncertain. Listen closely to what your doctor tells you, even writing down what he says, if necessary. Don't allow yourself to get sidetracked by irrelevant information, which will waste everybody's time. If you don't like a treatment she suggests, say so and ask for alternatives. And pay attention to your doctor's body language. When he starts glancing at his watch, he may be subtly telling you that he's running late.

Bring a notebook to your appointment and take notes. It's easy to forget some minor detail during a visit, so jot down anything that you think might be important. Some doctors may even allow you to tape-record the visit—just make sure to ask first. Anything you do to help you recall the information will spare your doctor the aggravation of follow-up phone calls and questions later on.

Also, be sure to follow through on what your doctor tells you to do. If he asks you to get a blood test, do so promptly. If she asks you to take a medication, take it exactly as she specifies. It's upsetting to doctors when patients ignore their directions.

Finally, be polite but firm. Doctors are more likely to dismiss an angry patient who becomes rude and hostile than one who is unemotional and assertive. You'll be more likely to be heard if you present yourself in a calm and professional manner. And remember to pay your bill on time. Prompt payment is part of your end of the bargain and will ensure good treatment at later visits.

All good relationships take effort on the part of both people in order to make things work. As the patient, you have to do your part to ensure a smooth relationship with your doctor. Keep in mind that the doctors you work with will be the same ones you see through the years as you continue to manage and monitor your thyroid disease. A strong and trusting relationship will help ensure that you stay healthy.

CHAPTER 4

Hypothyroidism

You sleep eight hours a night, but you still feel sluggish. You haven't changed your diet, but you're gaining weight. To top it off, you're feeling achy and depressed. It's easy to blame these symptoms on a busy lifestyle or advancing age, but for millions of people—especially women—your thyroid is the culprit. Hypothyroidism develops when your thyroid isn't producing enough thyroid hormone. In this chapter, you'll learn all about this type of thyroid disease—from being diagnosed to seeking treatment.

What Is Hypothyroidism?

Millions of people suffer from some form of thyroid disease. The vast majority—approximately 80 percent—have an underactive thyroid, or what is called hypothyroidism. According to the AACE, hypothyroidism affects about 10 percent of all women and 3 percent of men. Studies suggest that approximately 13 million Americans are undiagnosed.

Several factors can cause the thyroid to reduce its production of thyroid hormone. Here in the United States, the most common cause of hypothyroidism is an autoimmune disorder called Hashimoto's thyroiditis, in which the body launches an internal attack on its own healthy thyroid tissues, destroying the gland's ability to produce thyroid hormone. (You'll learn more about Hashimoto's in Chapter 6.) Hypothyroidism is also more common with aging. By age sixty, 17 percent of all women and 9 percent of men will have an underactive thyroid.

Around the world, the condition is caused primarily by a deficiency of iodine, a mineral found in saltwater, that the body uses to produce thyroid hormone. But with the introduction of iodized salt in the United States in the 1920s, iodine deficiency is practically unheard of in this country.

 Fact

Primary hypothyroidism refers to an underactive thyroid caused by a deficiency in thyroid hormone. Central hypothyroidism is a term that describes a reduction in thyroid hormone caused by problems with the pituitary gland. Although the causes differ, treatment is usually the same.

In some cases, hypothyroidism may be linked to other medical conditions or caused by a medication. For instance, people who have been treated with RAI to treat hyperthyroidism often develop hypothyroidism. Those who take medications such as lithium, prednisone, and propranolol are also vulnerable to hypothyroidism. In addition, anyone who has undergone thyroid surgery, also called thyroidectomy, or radiation to the neck or upper chest is likely to develop an underactive thyroid.

Of course, not everyone who gets older or takes these medications will develop hypothyroidism. But your risk does go up if you have other risk factors, including:

- A family history of thyroid problems
- A personal history of endocrine disease, including diabetes
- Illnesses or injuries involving the hypothalamus and/or the pituitary gland
- A personal or family history of autoimmune illness
- Recent pregnancy and delivery

- Illnesses such as chronic fatigue immune deficiency syndrome or fibromyalgia

Regardless of what triggers an underactive thyroid, the end result is the same: hypothyroidism causes all your body functions to slow down. This total-body slowdown produces signs and symptoms that will eventually become apparent.

What Hypothyroidism Looks Like

When your thyroid first starts to produce less thyroid hormone, you won't know it. It's rare to have any symptoms initially, and you may feel perfectly fine. Over time, however, as your metabolism begins to slow, you may start to notice that you are sluggish and fatigued.

Gradually, the condition begins to take its toll on your entire body, slowing everything from your heart rate to your digestion. Below are some of the most notable symptoms of hypothyroidism. Keep in mind that you may not have all these symptoms.

Weight Gain

For many people, the most disturbing symptom of hypothyroidism is unexplained weight gain, which occurs—ironically—even as your appetite shrinks. If you've been trying to lose weight, you might find it has become impossible, no matter how little you eat or how much exercise you do. In fact, even your best efforts to eat less may be met with weight gain.

Essential

Your thyroid gland is only one factor influencing your basal metabolic rate (BMR). BMR is also affected by genetics, the amount of exercise you do, and your body's fat and muscle composition. Those who exercise more have a faster BMR, as do people who have more muscle. BMR can also be affected by illnesses such as diabetes.

The weight you're gaining, however, is initially the result of swelling and not the accumulation of fat. As the kidneys retain more water and sodium, more water is left to circulate in the body, causing tissues to swell and weight to climb. Eventually, the body will also accumulate fat. Most of the time, it will top off at no more than ten to twenty pounds—just enough to set off alarm bells and make it hard to squeeze into your jeans. Occasionally, people with hypothyroidism will gain even more weight.

Foggy Mind

Forgetfulness is often a by-product of our busy and stress-filled lives. But in people who have hypothyroidism, the mind may feel similarly strained. Efforts to concentrate and focus may feel overwhelming, and your memory may become shaky and unreliable. Some people call this brain fog. As a result, it can be difficult to follow simple directions or perform your job. This problem can also slow your reaction time, which can affect your driving ability.

Depression

It's normal for everyone to experience an occasional bout of the blues, especially if you're going through a difficult time. But in people who have depression, feelings of emptiness, helplessness, and hopelessness may linger for no real apparent reason. As a result, you may lose interest in activities that normally brought you great joy. Such feelings are a normal symptom of hypothyroidism and generally go away once the hypothyroidism is treated.

Dry Skin, Hair, and Nails

It's bad enough that low thyroid function is making you tired, swollen, and depressed. Unfortunately, a sluggish thyroid can take a toll on your appearance, too. Skin may become pale and dry, and even crack. Hair may become dry and brittle. Some people may notice that they are losing more hair than normal, and that hair loss is occurring elsewhere on their body, too. A common place to lose hair is at the outer part of your eyebrows. At the same time, fingernails may become dry and brittle and develop grooves that cause the surface to become uneven.

Sluggish Gastrointestinal Tract

Thyroid hormones play a role in the way your body breaks down food and moves it through the gastrointestinal tract. That's because your digestive tract is lined with muscles that contract in order to propel the digested food. When you become deficient in thyroid hormone, this digestive process slows down. As the propulsion of food into the bowel slows, you may notice that you are frequently constipated.

Irregular Menstruation and Difficulty with Pregnancy

Women who have hypothyroidism may notice that their periods have become heavier and more frequent. Some women may stop ovulating, making it difficult to get pregnant. It may also be difficult to retain a pregnancy: Six of every 100 miscarriages are the result of hypothyroidism.

Alert

It's easy to mistake hypothyroidism for premenstrual syndrome (PMS). The two conditions have similar symptoms—fatigue, depression, bloating, and weight gain, among them. Having an underactive thyroid can make your PMS symptoms worse. If you suffer from bothersome PMS, ask to have your thyroid checked. Treating your thyroid problems usually lessens your PMS, too.

Swollen Thyroid Gland

In some people with hypothyroidism, the gland may actually become enlarged, creating a condition called a goiter. Some people can see this enlargement by performing the neck check. You may also notice that your voice is hoarse as the swollen gland presses against your vocal cords. In some cases, you may experience coughing, difficulty breathing, and trouble swallowing.

Impaired Heart Function

Hypothyroidism causes your pulse to slow as your heart rate decreases. In addition, your heart may weaken, and fluid can seep into the heart muscle, causing it to swell. You may also experience an increase in your blood pressure. As a result of this slowdown in activity, your heart is forced to work harder to get oxygen and nutrients throughout your body. This can put you at risk for heart failure, a potentially life-threatening condition.

Other Changes

Hypothyroidism causes myriad other bodily functions to change, too. For instance, you may notice that you are extra sensitive to cold temperatures, and that your hands feel cold. You may notice that you are less interested in sex or that your allergies seem worse. You may also experience frequent headaches and notice that your muscles are achy, tender, and stiff. Any cuts, bruises, and infections you suffer may take longer than normal to heal.

Blood tests may reveal other health problems associated with your underactive thyroid. For instance, you may develop high cholesterol, a problem that can lead to heart disease if left untreated. You may also develop anemia or low red blood cell counts. In hypothyroidism, the anemia is typically the result of a deficiency of iron in the blood.

Alert

Women who have hypothyroidism have another reason to quit smoking. Studies show that women who smoke have higher levels of LDL, the bad cholesterol, as well as higher total cholesterol levels, both risks for heart disease. The smokers also had more muscle problems. Cigarette smoking apparently impairs the secretion and action of thyroid hormone.

Hypothyroidism also impacts how your body responds to its environment. Medications you take, for example, may produce more pronounced side effects. Some people, for instance, become more sensitive to stimulants like pseudoephedrine, which is often in cold remedies.

In some cases, it may take years for any symptoms of hypothyroidism to emerge. When they do, it's easy to mistake them for other health problems or life situations. It isn't until a thyroid test is done that a deficiency in thyroid hormone can be properly identified as the root of the problem.

Without treatment, all these symptoms may worsen over time. And if it goes untreated long enough, hypothyroidism can be deadly. The good news is, treatment is readily available and can quickly restore the thyroid to its proper function.

Making the Diagnosis

Treatment for hypothyroidism quickly improves your symptoms, but treatment is possible only if you're properly diagnosed. So if you suspect you have hypothyroidism, it's important to get diagnosed promptly.

To find out whether you are truly deficient in thyroid hormone, your doctor should perform a thorough physical exam and order a blood test. In some cases, the results of your blood test will make it clear that you have hypothyroidism. But in other cases, the results may be less revealing.

In any case, a doctor should also take into account the signs and symptoms that you are experiencing, and work toward getting you properly diagnosed, even if it isn't hypothyroidism causing your problems. After all, many of these symptoms do overlap with other medical conditions such as depression, chronic fatigue syndrome, and fibromyalgia.

To figure out whether you have hypothyroidism, your doctor will want to know your health history as well as that of your family. He should engage you in a conversation about your health and probe into your health status. What symptoms are you concerned about? How are your mood and energy level? Do you notice any swelling or changes in your voice?

Your physician will also perform a physical exam. He may check your fingernails, your complexion, and your pulse. He should also perform a hands-on check of the thyroid gland to see if it is enlarged.

During the visit, be sure to share details about your health, including any medications you may be taking and any recent illnesses. Don't be shy about discussing your lack of libido or your recent bouts of depression. Although these details may seem embarrassing to you, they are actually signs and symptoms of disease that can assist your doctor in making a proper diagnosis.

Blood Tests

One of the most important things your doctor will do is order blood tests to figure out if you have hypothyroidism. Blood tests are critical in determining whether your thyroid is the cause of your symptoms. It's also a relatively simple process. What does get tricky is making sense of the alphabet soup that comes with the lab results.

TSH Levels

For most doctors, the most telling measure of all is the level of TSH in your blood. As you might recall, TSH is the hormone released by the pituitary gland that tells the thyroid gland to release more hormones. Higher-than-normal levels of TSH reveal that your pituitary is trying to stimulate the thyroid gland to release more thyroid hormone.

The American College of Clinical Endocrinologists currently considers normal levels of TSH to be in the range of 0.3 milliunits per deciliter (mIU/dL) to 3.0 mIU/dL—a change made in November 2002, when the range was narrowed from the previous range of 0.5 mIU/dL to 5.0 mIU/dL. The new, more stringent definition of normal has paved the way for more diagnoses of hypo- and hyperthyroidism. Anything above that range might be considered hypothyroidism, depending on other factors. Measures below it might be hyperthyroidism.

Although TSH levels are considered the best gauge of thyroid function, there are times when this measure is less than ideal. For instance, measuring TSH assumes that the pituitary gland is healthy and functioning properly. But if the pituitary gland has a tumor, it may be incapable of producing enough TSH. Deficiencies in TSH may also be caused by damage to the hypothalamus brought on by an injury, tumor, or stroke. In these cases, the TSH level may be inappropriately normal, even when levels of thyroid hormone are low.

In addition, the time of day that your blood is drawn makes a difference. TSH tends to be in the midrange in the early morning, drops at noon, then rises at night.

Total T4 and Free T4

Total T4 is just that—a measure of all the T4 in your blood, including the T4 that is bound to protein and unavailable to body cells for use. In fact, the bulk of the T4 released by your thyroid is bound to proteins.

Alert

A good thyroid doctor will rely on more than just the TSH test as a way to diagnose hypo- or hyperthyroidism. The TSH test, after all, reveals only part of the picture; that is, how much the pituitary gland is egging on the thyroid gland for more hormone. More comprehensive testing will involve tests for free T3 and free T4—the actual amount of available thyroid hormone.

Although testing for total T4 has been used in the past to diagnose hypothyroidism, today it is considered a less useful tool. That's because the amount of total T4 can be affected by the amount of binding proteins in the blood. The amount of protein is influenced by medical conditions such as certain types of liver and kidney diseases as well as by pregnancy. Nonetheless, low levels of total T4 can often suggest that you have hypothyroidism.

A more useful diagnostic tool is the free T4 test. This test measures the unbound T4 in the blood, which is called free thyroxine. Too little of it is a sign of hypothyroidism.

If your doctor decides to test free T4, he should use a lab that uses the equilibrium dialysis method, which involves separating the free hormone from the bound version. Free T4 is the thyroid hormone available to enter body cells, where it can be converted into T3, the active form of thyroid hormone.

In patients who have hypothyroidism, free T4 levels are rarely lower than normal. Patients with hypothyroidism, especially mild hypothyroidism, usually have an elevated TSH with a low-normal free T4 because the TSH goes up before the free T4 does. Your doctor needs to consider the relationship between free T4 and TSH to see if there is a discrepancy that may suggest a problem.

Total T3 and Free T3

T3, also called triiodothyronine, is the active form of thyroid hormone. The total T3 in your blood is generally not an accurate measure of hypothyroidism, but may be used to diagnose hyperthyroidism.

Another test that is occasionally helpful for diagnosing hypothyroidism is one that measures the amount of free T3 in your body. Free T3 is the active form of triiodothyronine, the unbound version of the hormone that circulates in the blood. It is the active part of thyroid hormone produced by the conversion of T4 to T3. Again, if your doctor decides to measure free T3, he should use a lab that uses the equilibrium dialysis method for a more accurate measurement.

People who have hypothyroidism rarely have low levels of free T3. Most of the time, even in hypothyroidism, the body increases the enzymes that convert T4 to T3, so the free T3 remains normal.

An old way to indirectly measure free T4 and free T3 involves the resin T3 uptake test (RT_3U), an indirect measurement that estimates the amount of free T4 and free T3. This test tells you whether you have a lot of TBG, the protein that carries most of the T3 and T4 in your blood. RT_3U is inversely proportional to TBG levels; the more TBG you have, the lower your RT_3U levels will be.

High levels of TBG means there are more proteins available to bind T4 and T3, leaving less free T4 and free T3 in the blood. Elevated levels of TBG can be caused by pregnancy, estrogen, and oral contraceptives. Patients with altered levels of TBG do not have symptoms of hypo- or hyperthyroidism. In fact, if your doctor measures free T4 and free T3, the TBG alterations won't even be detected. For these reasons and others, the resin T3 uptake test is rarely used now and has been replaced by tests that directly measure free T4 and T3.

Thyroid Autoantibodies

When people get sick, the immune system produces antibodies to ward off the invading virus or bacteria. But in people who have an autoimmune condition, autoantibodies are produced to fight the patient's own body tissues, which for mysterious reasons are being treated as harmful invaders.

Unfortunately, the thyroid can be the target of an autoimmune attack. In the process, several antibodies may be produced. These substances are easily measured in the blood and serve as markers, or physical evidence, of a disease process.

An autoimmune attack on the thyroid gland often triggers the production of antithyroid peroxidase (TPO) antibodies. Anti-TPO antibodies wreak havoc by attacking parts of the thyroid cells that produce thyroid hormone. Testing for these anti-TPO antibodies has become the gold standard for detecting Hashimoto's disease. More than 80 percent of people with Hashimoto's will test positive for anti-TPO antibodies. Some doctors will test for anti-TPO antibodies even if other tests appear normal. If your anti-TPO antibodies are elevated, your hypothyroidism is probably caused by Hashimoto's thyroiditis.

Antithyroglobulin antibodies can also be found in Hashimoto's thyroiditis but are not as helpful as identifying the presence of anti-TPO antibodies and are not necessary to diagnose Hashimoto's thyroiditis. Similarly, some doctors may still order a test for antimicrosomal antibodies, which is a less specific test than the anti-TPO test. If you're already getting an anti-TPO test, then you do not need to be tested for antimicrosomal antibodies.

Normal Versus Abnormal Test Results

As you might have noticed, we have not described what constitutes high, low, or normal levels of most of these hormones and antibodies. So, you may wonder, how do I know if my measurements are normal or abnormal?

Ⅼ. Essential

> To check for hypo- or hyperthyroidism, Dr. Friedman places his hands just a touch below the patient's. If the patient's hands emit coldness, it's a sign of hypothyroidism. If they give off warmth, it's a sign of hyperthyroidism.

Exactly what constitutes normal varies considerably, depending on the lab your doctor uses. Different labs use different standards of measurement. And unlike some medical tests, which quickly reveal whether you do or don't have an infection—a strep culture is an example—thyroid hormone test results must be placed in proper context. This is known as the reference range, which some doctors may call the "normal" range.

A reference range is determined first by testing a large group of healthy people. Levels for this group are then taken together to create a range of what is considered healthy. The result of your test is then measured against a group that is similar to you in age, gender, and health status. For instance, pregnant women would have a different reference range than women of the same age who are not pregnant.

To find out if your hormone levels are normal, ask to see a copy of your lab report. On it, you should see a reference range for each particular test, along with your results.

Keep in mind that just because your test results fall into the reference range of what's considered healthy or "normal" doesn't mean that you do not have hypothyroidism. No group test can ever account for all individual differences in these lab tests, and different people will feel differently even if their test results are the same. That's why it's always important to discuss your test results with your doctor and to work toward uncovering the cause of your symptoms. If necessary, request a retest or ask that other tests be administered.

Putting It All Together

When it comes to diagnosing hypothyroidism, it's often important to perform several tests and to consider all the results before making a formal diagnosis. Although significantly elevated levels of TSH generally do indicate an underactive thyroid, a single test is sometimes not enough to determine whether you have hypothyroidism.

Instead, your doctor needs to consider all your test results as well as the physical exam of your thyroid and your self-reported symptoms. In some cases, all the tests may come back normal, despite the presence of numerous symptoms of hypothyroidism. If that's the case, you may need to be retested in six months. But if the tests do detect abnormalities, you may be diagnosed with some form of hypothyroidism. Here are some possible diagnoses, based on your lab results:

- **Mild (Subclinical) Hypothyroidism:** If you are mildly hypothyroid, you may have a normal free T3 test and a normal free T4 test. But your TSH levels may be high. See below for more discussion on this topic.
- **Hypothyroidism:** If you have hypothyroidism as a result of a deficiency in thyroid hormone, you will probably have a normal or low free T3 test, a low free T4 test, and elevated levels of TSH.
- **Hashimoto's Disease:** If you test positive for anti-TPO antibodies in addition to a normal or low free T3 test, low free T4 test, and high levels of TSH, your hypothyroidism may be caused by Hashimoto's thyroiditis. You may also have an enlarged thyroid gland.
- **Pituitary (Central) Hypothyroidism:** In rare cases, disease can affect your pituitary gland, making it unable to produce

enough TSH to stimulate your thyroid gland to produce enough thyroid hormone. As a result, your TSH levels will be low or low-normal, and your free T3 and free T4 levels may be low or normal. You may also have symptoms of pituitary dysfunction, including menstrual irregularities and low libido.

The Diagnosis Debate

Exactly how many people have hypothyroidism in the United States is unclear. The Colorado Thyroid Disease Prevalence Study in 2000 found that as many as 13 million people may not be properly diagnosed. A diagnosis also depends on where the reference range is set and what your doctor believes. Some doctors may diagnose you with hypothyroidism if your TSH levels are even slightly elevated, while others may not unless levels become significantly high.

To make matters even more complicated, TSH levels fluctuate and may vary with diet, medications, the time of day you have your blood drawn, and the time of year. For instance, during colder months, TSH levels naturally rise. It may also rise when you are taking medications such as lithium or eating too many soy products, which contain isoflavones that boost TSH. In addition, TSH drops in the early part of pregnancy and rises during the latter part.

The murky nature of diagnosing hypothyroidism has sparked some controversy in endocrine circles. According to the *New York Times,* the controversy erupted in January 2004, when a panel of experts from several organizations published a report in the *Journal of the American Medical Association.*

The group—made up of experts from the American Thyroid Association (ATA), the AACE, and the Endocrine Society—said it found no significant scientific evidence to treat patients with mild hypothyroidism, even if these patients were experiencing symptoms. The panel recommended against screening the population for thyroid disease, but suggested that doctors be on guard with high-risk patients, such as older women.

In response, the groups that sponsored the panel disagreed and published a rebuttal in the *Journal of Clinical Endocrinology &*

Metabolism. Proponents of more stringent testing have recommended lowering the upper limit of what is considered normal, so that more people who need treatment are properly diagnosed.

Still others take issue with the notion of a "normal" level of TSH. As Mary J. Shomon, a patient advocate and thyroid patient herself, said in the *Times* article, "What's normal for me may not be normal for you. We're patients, not lab values."

In any case, the debate over what's normal and what's not is far from over. But it may explain why some people have a hard time convincing their doctors that they do have hypothyroidism, even if their blood tests show values that could be considered abnormal.

Question

What is Wilson's syndrome?
Former physician E. Denis Wilson coined the term for a vague condition characterized by low body temperature and symptoms that resemble hypothyroidism. The American Thyroid Association (ATA) has dismissed the syndrome as having no scientific basis in fact and does not support the use of body temperature as a way to diagnose hypothyroidism. The condition is not to be confused with Wilson's disease, which is a rare genetic condition involving copper metabolism.

One result of this debate is the question of whether to treat people with mild or subclinical hypothyroidism. For patients, this situation has meant that people on the high end of the normal range provided by the laboratory—those with a TSH, say, of 3.0 to 5.0 mIU/dL, for instance—may not be treated for mild hypothyroidism, even in the face of uncomfortable symptoms. Some experts argue that there is no clear, compelling reason to treat these people before they develop true hypothyroidism. But other medical experts disagree and contend that treatment could help prevent the onset of hypothyroidism.

(*Note:* Dr. Friedman will treat a patient with a goiter and a positive anti-TPO test who has a TSH greater than 3.5 mIU/dL. He will also treat a patient who has no goiter and a negative anti-TPO test, with a TSH greater than 7.0 mIU/dL.)

If you happen to have subclinical hypothyroidism, you should discuss your options with your doctor. If you have no symptoms, you may be advised to adopt a wait-and-see approach, with more frequent testing to keep an eye on thyroid function. But if you are suffering from bothersome symptoms, you may need to explore your treatment options now. If your doctor is reluctant to treat you, you may want to consider switching to a doctor who is more apt to treat subclinical hypothyroidism.

The Importance of Treatment

Not treating hypothyroidism is simply not an option. Left untreated, hypothyroidism can cause serious complications such as high cholesterol—which can lead to heart disease—and infertility. In extreme cases, it can lead to coma or death.

Thyroid hormone is essential to your health, and if you've become hypothyroid for any reason, it is critical that you replace the missing hormone. Most people who develop hypothyroidism will have it for the rest of their life and will require thyroid hormone replacement. Chances are, you will be on your medication for life to compensate for your natural deficiency in thyroid hormone. You will also need to monitor the effect of your medication on a regular basis. Luckily, treatment is often quite successful at eliminating your symptoms and restoring your health. And once you've established the right dose for your body, the amount of monitoring will go down. Taking your pill will simply become a part of your daily routine.

Chapter 5

Treating Hypothyroidism

Now that you know your thyroid is underactive, you'll need to start treatment to restore the hormones you're missing. The key is pinpointing the appropriate dosage and understanding all the factors that can affect it. In this chapter, you'll learn what your drug options are, how to take your medication correctly, and what side effects and complications can result.

Drug Options

People who have hypothyroidism need thyroid hormone replacement, and they'll probably need it for the rest of their lives. Once the right dosage is established, thyroid hormone replacement works well and is safe and easily tolerated. You'll soon notice that your symptoms will ease up and your health will improve. Blood tests will reveal that your T4 and TSH levels are back to normal.

But sometimes, establishing the right dosage of thyroid hormone replacement can be tricky. It may take a few months before you and your doctor figure out the right amount. After all, what works for one patient with a similar profile may not always work for another. Working with your doctor, you will have to experiment with different dosages and get regular blood tests before you pin down the one that works for you.

You also need to make sure you are on the correct form of thyroid hormone replacement. These drugs come in different varieties and brands. You may fare better on one brand or type than you would on another, and it may take some time and experimenting before you figure out which one works best. In addition, you'll need to take and store these drugs correctly.

Synthetic T4

Most doctors today start their hypothyroid patients on synthetic T4. Although T3 is the active form of thyroid hormone, T4 is readily converted to T3 in body tissues. T4 is also the more stable form of thyroid hormone, which helps ensure that blood levels of thyroid hormone remain more even, so that you don't experience the highs and lows that come with taking T3.

The generic name of synthetic T4 is levothyroxine, which is sold under several brand names, the most popular being Synthroid. Although Synthroid was prescribed for years, it did not receive approval from the U.S. Food and Drug Administration until 2003. Since its debut in the 1950s, it had been considered an equivalent of natural hormone (Armour) and so was grandfathered in and spared the approval process required of new drugs. But concerns about potency and stability prompted the FDA to revisit all levothyroxine products and require their manufacturers to apply for approval as new drugs.

By 2004, Synthroid was the second most popular drug in the United States—behind Lipitor, the cholesterol-lowering agent—with more than 42 million prescriptions sold. Other brand names include Levoxyl, Unithroid, and Levothroid.

Some patients may prefer one brand over another, but all the brands are made of synthetic thyroxine. Like the real T4 that your body makes, synthetic T4 tends to remain in the blood for a long time, providing your body cells with a steady supply of thyroid hormone. If your doctor prescribes one brand for you, you should not switch to another brand without his knowledge. Also, ask your doctor to write "DAW" on your prescription. DAW stands for "dispense as written" and will help ensure that a generic is not substituted. If your pharmacist tries to switch your brand, you should insist on getting the drug you are prescribed.

Levothyroxine comes in different color-coded doses. The 50 mcg pill is white and contains no dye, so that people allergic to dyes have that option. Depending on the dosage you're prescribed, you may take the pills singly or in combination. In some cases, you may be able to cut a pill—they do have a line down the middle for easy cutting—and save some money and trips to the pharmacy.

L. Essential

Although the active ingredient in all the brands of levothyroxine is the same, different brands contain different fillers and are subject to their own quality controls. That's why it's best to find one brand you like and to stick with it.

For most patients with hypothyroidism, treatment with T4 alone is often successful and adequate. Once on T4, their TSH levels will drop to normal, and symptoms will disappear. But if symptoms don't fade, you may need to be treated with T3 as well.

Synthetic T3

As you probably recall, T3 is the active form of thyroid hormone. The synthetic form of T3 is used primarily to lessen the symptoms of hypothyroidism when preparing for whole-body scans, which require that you become hypothyroid. Synthetic T3 is called liothyronine and is sold under the brand name Cytomel.

Synthetic T3 works in the body for only a few hours, so you need to take several doses a day to derive its benefits. Taking T3 also disrupts the way your body naturally controls and regulates TSH levels. And if you take only T3, you will experience low T4 levels. In addition, taking too much T3 can stress the heart.

Still, some patients with hypothyroidism may require T3 if they continue to have symptoms of hypothyroidism even after their TSH levels normalize from the use of T4. Some experts contend that the presence of symptoms suggests that you are having trouble converting T4 into T3. Others dispute that notion and argue that the problem is really another health issue unrelated to the thyroid.

In any case, some doctors may prescribe T3 to address the lingering symptoms. The science on the use of T3 is mixed: Some studies have suggested that patients do better when they take both T4 and T3. But other studies have found no difference in patients receiving T4 alone versus a combination of T3 and T4.

It's possible, but not proven, that patients with low blood levels of free T3 may benefit from T3 treatment. It is also possible that patients who do not fare well on T4 alone may have low levels of T3 in the brain, which cannot be detected without a brain biopsy.

Alert

It's dangerous to take Cytomel—or any other thyroid hormone for that matter—as a way to lose weight. Too much thyroid hormone certainly can rev up the metabolism and result in weight loss. But many people without a thyroid disorder who take thyroid hormone gain weight because their appetite increases. Taking thyroid hormone can also put you into a state of hyperthyroidism, which can cause heart problems and osteoporosis.

In his practice, Dr. Friedman tends to start patients on T4 by itself and adjust the dosage until their TSH is between 0.5 and 2 mIU/dL. If the patient still has symptoms—despite normal TSH levels—Dr. Friedman might add low doses of T3. (Although Cytomel is taken two or three times a day, patients can use a compounding pharmacy that will make a slow-release T3 that is taken once a day. Unfortunately, most insurance companies will not cover the cost of compounded medications.) Dr. Friedman is more inclined to treat patients with T3 if initial tests showed they had low levels of free T3 in their blood.

If they are given both T4 and T3, he checks to make sure their blood levels of free T4 and free T3 are in the higher end of normal. When patients are on this type of combination treatment, they are likely to have lower levels of TSH since T3 suppresses the TSH.

Synthetic T4 and T3

Some patients who need T3 may be given a drug that combines both T4 and T3. This combination drug is called liotrix and sold under the brand name Thyrolar. The ratio of T3 to T4 in Thyrolar is 1 to 4. If you are prescribed Thyrolar, make sure to store it in the refrigerator.

The disadvantage of Thyrolar is that the T3 to T4 ratio is fixed. If your doctor gives you T3 and T4 separately, she can adjust that ratio to better match your needs.

Desiccated Thyroid Drugs

In the years before synthetic T4 was available, people who had hypothyroidism relied on desiccated thyroid hormone replacement to restore their missing hormones. In fact, Armour, the most well-known brand, was the only thyroid hormone drug on the market for the first half of the twentieth century. Today, it remains a popular treatment despite the use of synthetic thyroid hormone, with almost $2.5 million in sales in 2004, according to *Drug Topics*, an online pharmacy publication.

These treatments are made from hormones extracted from the thyroid glands of pigs. They contain both T4 and T3 and are sold under several brand names, Armour being the most popular. Other brands include Bio-Throid, Westhroid, and Nature-Throid. These medications are particularly appealing to patients who prefer using "natural" products to synthetic ones.

Although it has not been proven, some experts believe that desiccated thyroid hormone contains other hormones or factors made by the thyroid, which are not found in synthetic hormones.

Some conventional doctors are more resistant to using desiccated thyroid hormone in their patients, believing that synthetic products are best. But in reality, some patients do better on these products than they do on the synthetic ones. If you are on synthetic hormones and have a normal TSH (0.5–2.0 mIU/dL) but are still not feeling well, you should discuss the possibility of trying natural hormone therapy.

Some people are concerned about the consistency of the different batches of these products. Since the thyroid hormones come from pigs, it is quite possible that the amount of thyroid hormone in the gland of each animal will vary somewhat. On the other hand, most manufacturers do take steps to ensure consistency. Forest Pharmaceuticals, Inc., which makes Armour, for one, says it tests both the powder and the finished tablet to ensure that the amount of hormone is consistent. Any inconsistency that might occur is usually so slight as to be insignificant.

Essential

If you have trouble convincing your doctor that you should try natural hormone therapy, consider finding a more open-minded physician who will let you give it a try. Armour is also much cheaper than synthetic thyroid hormone.

With patients who do not improve on T4 treatment alone or combined T4 and T3 therapy, Dr. Friedman will sometimes switch to a natural treatment, usually Armour, plus synthetic T4. He adds T4 to the regimen to make up for the higher T3 to T4 ratio found in Armour. When he tests them, he looks for free T4 and free T3 in the upper ranges of normal.

Taking Drugs Correctly

When you first start taking thyroxine, some doctors may start you on the lowest possible dose. Other doctors (including Dr. Friedman) will recommend starting on a full replacement dosage unless you are elderly or have heart problems. The advantage of starting on a full replacement dose is that you will feel better sooner. The dose you take will be based on several factors, including your age, weight, the cause of your hypothyroidism, and whether you are taking other medications. A rough guide is the dose of T4 in micrograms you will need is equal to your weight in kilograms times 1.6. One kilogram equals 2.2 pounds.

In general, the more you weigh, the higher the dose. And if you are older, you will probably start on a low dose so that your body can adjust. Drugs generally move more slowly in older people, so you may wind up staying on a low dose. But if you do need more medication, your doctor will probably increase it very slowly.

The cause of your hypothyroidism also may dictate the dose you receive. If you have Hashimoto's disease or mild hypothyroidism, for instance, some doctors believe your thyroid may still be making some hormone, and you probably need a lower dose. Other doctors recommend full replacement even for mild hypothyroidism. But if you have had your thyroid removed, you will often need a higher dose to make up for the missing hormone. In any case, taking too much thyroxine can trigger symptoms of hyperthyroidism—anxiety, restlessness, and a rapid heartbeat.

Question

Are generic thyroid drugs as good as brand-name ones?
Although doctors almost always prescribe brand name, some pharmacies—or health maintenance organizations (HMOs)—may actually try to give you a generic version. The American Thyroid Association (ATA) recommends that you stick with brand names whenever possible since generics may not be consistent from one refill to the next. Always check that you were dispensed the brand you were prescribed.

Whatever thyroid hormone replacement drug you wind up taking, it's critical that you take it correctly and follow your doctor's orders closely. Becoming familiar with your thyroid hormone drug—which drugs and foods affect it, how to store it, and when to expect to feel better—can make a big difference in how well the medication works for you. Here are some important facts to know.

Be Consistent

The key to successful thyroid hormone replacement is taking it every day—every single day. One of the most important things you can do to ensure that you remember to take your pill is to take it at the same time every day. Most doctors recommend taking your pill first thing in the morning. Link it to another daily habit such as brushing your teeth or just before taking your morning shower. Some people find it easier to remember by keeping their pills in containers marked by the days of the week.

If you miss a dose, don't panic. T4 tends to remain in your blood for a long time. Simply take your pill when you remember it. If you forgot to take your pill yesterday, you can take one pill (the forgotten one) in the morning and one in the evening. It's best to not take two pills at once. Or, you can probably skip the one you missed. If you're concerned, call your doctor or pharmacist and ask what you should do.

It's also important to take the brand that you are prescribed. Although each brand contains the same active ingredients, some of the filler ingredients may differ and can affect the way your body absorbs the drug. If you do want to try another drug, you must do so under a doctor's supervision and get your TSH tested and dosage adjusted, if necessary.

Alert

Always take your thyroid medication with a full glass of water. Depending on the brand you take, some tablets may expand and get stuck in your throat, causing gagging or choking.

People who take drugs that contain T3 should talk to their doctors about taking their drugs at different times of the day. T3 is a faster-acting drug that loses its effect after just a few hours. Taking it two or three times a day can sometimes help even out your hormone levels.

Give It Time

You've been taking your pill every day for three weeks now, but you're still feeling lousy. You may be wondering why the drug isn't working. Meanwhile, your sister noticed improvements in just two weeks. What's going on?

In reality, the impact of thyroid medication varies from one person to the next. For some people, the effects may kick in in just two weeks. In others, it might take six weeks before the drug starts to work and you notice any significant improvements. In any case, around four to six weeks, your doctor will do another set of thyroid tests. If your TSH levels are still high—or they've gone too low—your doctor will need to adjust your dosage accordingly.

In some cases, it can take months before you and your doctor pinpoint the best dosage. Be patient. Finding the best dose is a matter of trial and error. You will eventually find the right dosage.

Store It Properly

Most people stash their medications in the bathroom cabinet, where they're easily accessible in the morning or evening. But in reality, the bathroom isn't always the best place for drugs that need to be at room temperature, which includes most thyroid medications.

Levothyroxine, for instance, is sensitive to heat. Heat and steam from several showers can raise the temperature in a bathroom cabinet enough to affect the potency of the drugs stored there. Other storage places you need to beware of include kitchen cupboards near the stove or dishwasher, the glove compartment of your car, or a counter or window ledge that sits in direct sunlight.

Instead, store the drug at room temperature in cabinets that are removed from heat and light. The only drug for hypothyroidism that requires refrigeration is liotrix (Thyrolar).

Watch What You Eat

The foods you eat and medicines you take can have a big effect on how well your body absorbs your thyroid medication. Ideally, you should take your pill on an empty stomach since food can delay absorption. It's best to wait an hour after you take your pill before eating. But if you need to eat something before taking your thyroid drug, do that every day, and discuss it with your doctor. The key is to be consistent. Varying it will make absorption erratic and cause hormone levels to be irregular.

L. Essential

Some experts believe that certain foods, eaten raw, can promote thyroid problems by blocking the thyroid's uptake of iodine. These foods are known as goitrogens and include items such as broccoli, cabbage, kale, cauliflower, Brussels sprouts, and turnips. In reality, however, most goitrogens do not cause thyroid problems unless eaten in large quantities.

Certain foods and supplements can inhibit your body's absorption of thyroid medications, too. A diet rich in fiber, for example, may decrease the amount of thyroid medication that your body absorbs. If you're already eating a high-fiber diet at the time you start taking thyroid replacement, your body will settle into the proper dosage with the fiber taken into account. But if you decide to start eating a high-fiber diet after starting your thyroid drug, be sure to let your doctor know. You may need a higher dose of thyroid medication.

In addition, some substances and minerals in food can inhibit absorption of thyroid medications. These substances should not be ingested at the same time you take your thyroid drug. Foods and supplements that inhibit absorption include:

- Calcium supplements and calcium-fortified foods
- Iron supplements

- Soy foods and other foods that contain isoflavones
- Antacids that contain either calcium or aluminum hydroxide

Taking calcium or iron is especially problematic. If you must eat these foods or take these supplements, make sure to wait at least one hour after taking your thyroid medication before doing so. Spacing them out will reduce the likelihood that these foods and supplements will affect your thyroid treatment.

Be Wary of Drug Combinations

Foods and supplements aren't the only substances that can impact the way your thyroid hormone replacement works. Certain drugs can impact the effectiveness of your thyroid treatment, too. At the same time, thyroid hormone can have an effect on how these drugs work. That's why it's critical that you tell your doctor all the medications you are taking before he puts you on a thyroid drug.

Here is a partial list of the kinds of drugs that can affect your thyroid medication:

- **Cholesterol-lowering Medications:** Drugs that reduce cholesterol levels, such as Colestid and Questran, bind thyroid hormones and make them less effective.
- **Diabetes Drugs:** Diabetics who rely on insulin or sulfonylureas may notice that these treatments are more or less effective when they start taking thyroid medications.
- **Antidepressants:** When taken with thyroid hormone replacement, the therapeutic and toxic effects of tricyclic antidepressants may be increased. If taken with a selective serotonin reuptake inhibitor (SSRI) such as Prozac or Zoloft, your thyroid medication may become more or less effective.
- **Anticoagulants:** Medications such as warfarin (Coumadin) that are used to prevent blood clotting—known as blood thinners—can sometimes become more potent in the presence of thyroid medications.

- **Estrogen:** Contraceptives and hormone replacement therapy that contain estrogen may decrease the amount of thyroid hormone in your body and require you to take a higher dose.
- **Anticonvulsants:** Taking thyroid hormone replacement with drugs used to treat convulsions, such as Dilantin, can speed up the metabolism of the thyroid medication.
- **Gastrointestinal Medications:** Antacids that contain aluminum or magnesium, sucralfate (Carafate), and simethicone (GasX) can all affect the way your body absorbs thyroid hormone replacement.
- **Beta-blockers:** People who have high blood pressure, heart failure, or previous heart attacks may take drugs called beta-blockers. The potency of certain beta-blockers such as metoprolol (Lopressor) or propranolol (Inderal) may be reduced when you start taking a thyroid drug.

Other drugs that warrant mention include aspirin, steroids, amphetamines, theophylline (for asthma), and medications used to reduce appetite or lose weight. The effectiveness of all these medications may be affected when you start taking thyroid hormone replacement.

Obviously, the list of drugs that interact with thyroid medications is a lengthy one. Again, that's why it's critical that you tell your doctor about *all* the medications and supplements you are taking. You should also tell your doctor about any pre-existing medical conditions. While it doesn't necessarily mean that you'll have to stop taking these other drugs, it might mean that you need to adjust your dosage of one or both medications accordingly.

Life changes and disruptions in your habits and routines can also affect how well your thyroid medication works, even after you've figured out your dosage and been on it for a while. Bouts of stress, starting a high-fiber diet, or going on birth control pills, for instance, can all increase your need for more thyroid medication.

If you notice that your medication no longer seems to be working and your symptoms of hypothyroidism have returned, talk to your doctor. By doing some detective work, she may be able to pinpoint the reasons why your medication has become less effective. She'll also be able to adjust your dose to a level that does work.

Alert

If you'd like a listing of drugs that can affect your thyroid medication, check on the Internet for the individual medications. Many, such as Synthroid (*www.synthroid.com*) and Armour (*www.armourthyroid .com*), have their own Web sites, produced by their manufacturers . You can also find information on the National Library of Medicine Web site at *www.nlm.nih.gov*. But don't let the list alarm you. Most interactions are mild.

Side Effects and Complications

Luckily, drugs for hypothyroidism tend not to cause many side effects. The main problem with taking thyroid replacement occurs when you take too little or too much of the drug. Too much, and you could become hyperthyroid, which means you'll feel jittery, anxious, and short of breath, and have trouble sleeping. You may also be at risk for osteoporosis since you're speeding up the turnover of bone. Too little, and you'll continue experiencing the symptoms of hypothyroidism. The key to avoiding that problem is finding the perfect dosage, which is a process of trial and error.

Although rare, some people do notice side effects from taking thyroid hormone replacement. Some women, for instance, may notice changes in their menstrual periods. Occasionally, people may have an allergic reaction to the dyes in thyroid medications. Other possible side effects include:

- Weight loss
- Diarrhea

- Fever
- Hair loss
- Headache
- Irritability
- Leg cramps
- Nausea and vomiting
- Tremors
- Insomnia

Such side effects are a nuisance but are not considered serious unless they persist. If you experience chest pain or an irregular heartbeat, however, you should contact your doctor immediately. Other side effects that warrant immediate medical attention include difficulty breathing; excessive sweating; or swelling in the ankles, feet, and legs.

Essential

Most women are told to steer clear of medications while pregnant. Though this is generally a good idea, you should always continue to take your thyroid hormone replacement. Not only is the medication safe, but your body will need it to supply the growing fetus with thyroid hormone. The best thing to do is to tell your doctor ahead of time if you are trying to conceive and to let her know as soon as you do get pregnant. Your doctor may want to increase your dosage.

In people who take drugs that contain T3, the side effects are the same. Too much T3 can cause anxiety, insomnia, and a rapid heartbeat. The side effects may be most apparent shortly after you take T3, when your body gets its first jolt of the hormone.

Hashimoto's Thyroiditis

Autoimmune problems can affect virtually any part of the body, and the thyroid gland is no exception. When an autoimmune problem attacks the thyroid, the result is Hashimoto's thyroiditis. Today, Hashimoto's is the most common form of thyroiditis and the leading cause of hypothyroidism in the United States. In this chapter, you'll learn about causes, symptoms, diagnosis, and treatment of Hashimoto's, as well as the other forms of thyroiditis.

About Autoimmune Diseases

In healthy people, the immune system works like a vigilant defense squad, always on the lookout for foreign invaders like bacteria and viruses that threaten your health. Once invaded, the immune system goes to work, generating substances called antibodies, which go on the attack against the invaders, or antigens. The white blood cells work feverishly to destroy the invaders and bring about healing.

In someone who has an autoimmune disease, these white blood cells are mysteriously summoned for no apparent reason, and the body mistakenly treats normal healthy tissue as something foreign. The body then begins to produce antibodies against the perceived invader. Antibodies produced in an autoimmune disease are known as autoantibodies. In people with Hashimoto's, the most common antibodies are the thyroid peroxidase antibodies (TPOAb). These are the same antibodies that cause Graves' disease, which we will discuss in Chapter 9.

Fact

Though they may occur simultaneously, Hashimoto's thyroiditis is not the same thing as Hashimoto's encephalopathy, a rare autoimmune disease in which antibodies attack neurons in the brain. The same antibodies—anti-TPO—are involved in both conditions, and both conditions were identified by the same doctor. With Hashimoto's encephalopathy, you may experience dementia, tremors, headaches, and partial paralysis. It is sometimes mistaken for Alzheimer's, but it is treatable with steroids. Fortunately, Hashimoto's encephalopathy is rare.

An autoimmune attack can occur in various organs and body systems, each causing its own disease and constellation of symptoms. Antibodies that attack connective tissue cause systemic lupus erythematosus. Those that harm the joints cause rheumatoid arthritis. Those that target the tissues of the thyroid gland cause Hashimoto's thyroiditis, named for the Japanese surgeon who first identified the disease in 1912.

The Details of Hashimoto's

Hashimoto's disease is the most common cause of hypothyroidism in the United States and affects approximately 14 million Americans. It is also the most common cause of goiter in this country. The disease occurs most frequently in women between the ages of thirty and fifty.

Hashimoto's disease is also called chronic lymphocytic thyroiditis because of the lymphocytes—disease-fighting white blood cells—that are found in the thyroid tissue. The disease is characterized by inflammation of the thyroid gland. In many cases, people who have Hashimoto's will go on to develop hypothyroidism.

Causes

No one knows exactly what causes the body's immune system to turn against itself in Hashimoto's—or any other autoimmune disorder for that matter. Like most other autoimmune conditions, Hashimoto's tends to run in families. You might have a mother who has type I diabetes, an aunt who has lupus, and a sister who has Hashimoto's.

Because autoimmune problems are much more prevalent in women, some experts think that hormones somehow play a role in the disease process. But as of now, no one knows for sure how reproductive hormones might promote autoimmune disorders.

Some experts suspect that environmental factors are at play, too. Stress, viruses, infections, pollution, bacteria, and other influences may spur on the development of autoimmune disease. But again, these are theories, and the exact cause of any autoimmune disease remains a mystery. Most researchers believe that it's a combination of genetics and environmental factors that cause Hashimoto's.

Symptoms

Initially, many people with Hashimoto's have no symptoms at all. But over time, they may develop a goiter. Some patients may notice the goiter as a painless swelling at the base of their neck. Sometimes, this swelling can make it difficult to swallow or breathe.

After a while, as more thyroid tissue is destroyed, you may develop symptoms of hypothyroidism. Not everyone with Hashimoto's or the anti-TPOs gets hypothyroidism, but if you do, you may notice that you are more tired than usual, and that you're frequently forgetful. You may be especially sensitive to the cold, and your skin, nails, and hair may become dry. If you are a woman, your menstrual periods may become heavier and more painful. And if you're trying to get pregnant, you may suffer recurrent miscarriages.

Less commonly, Hashimoto's may initially trigger hyperthyroidism, a condition sometimes called Hashitoxicosis. As the thyroid cells are destroyed, large amounts of stored thyroid hormone are released into the bloodstream, causing a rapid heartbeat and feelings of anxiety and nervousness. Then, as the hormone dissipates, your body returns to normal functioning for a while, before going into a state of hypothyroidism when the thyroid isn't able to produce enough thyroid hormone. Gloria remembers how her hypothyroidism began with a bout of hyperthyroidism:

> Gloria was in her thirties when she started having severe pain in her lower neck. She was rapidly losing weight and having bouts of crying for no apparent reason. She didn't feel like herself and felt so out of control that she went to see a psychiatrist, who referred her to an endocrinologist. The doctor found hot nodules—the kind that take up RAI—which indicated an overactive thyroid gland. But over time, the nodules turned cold, and eventually, she was deficient in thyroid hormone and put on Synthroid. Thirty years later, she is still taking Synthroid and has her thyroid checked every year.

Diagnosis and Treatment

The good news is Hashimoto's is relatively easy to diagnose. Blood tests are done to look for specific antibodies, namely, thyroid peroxidase antibodies (TPOAb) and, in some cases, thyroglobulin antibodies (TgAb). TPOAb attack an enzyme called thyroid peroxidase inside the thyroid cells, which is involved in the uptake of iodine to produce thyroid hormone. TgAb destroy thyroglobulin, the protein that stores thyroid hormone, and disrupts the process of hormone production. In general, if TPO antibodies are measured, TgAb do not need to be measured. Oddly enough, the same antibodies that cause Hashimoto's can also cause Graves' disease.

Studies have suggested that about 10 percent of the population has low levels of these autoantibodies in their blood, but most of these people have no symptoms or health problems. In people with Hashimoto's, however, the levels are significantly higher.

In addition to autoantibodies, your doctor will probably test your TSH levels. Elevated levels of TSH are a key indicator of hypothyroidism. Even a slight reduction in the amount of thyroid hormone being produced can cause your TSH levels to rise. Some people with normal levels of TSH, however, can still have autoantibodies in their blood.

Ľ.. Essential

> Not everyone who has Hashimoto's has a goiter, and not all patients have symptoms of hypothyroidism. What everyone does have in common is the presence of antibodies that destroy thyroid tissue.

Some doctors may do a fine needle aspiration (FNA) of your thyroid, especially if you have a nodule as well as a goiter. The cells removed from your thyroid gland are then examined under a microscope for the presence of abnormal white blood cells. An FNA is rarely done except in cases that are difficult to diagnose and to rule out the possibility of cancer.

In people who have Hashimoto's that starts off with hyperthyroidism, the disease can be harder to diagnose. Since some of the same autoantibodies are also present in Graves' disease, your doctor may mistakenly diagnose you with Graves'. One way to distinguish Graves' from Hashimoto's is with a free T4 test. In people with Hashitoxicosis, levels of free T4 will gradually diminish as the thyroid hormone dissipates.

In some cases, an RAI uptake test can also help confirm Hashimoto's. This test involves ingesting a small amount of RAI. Hours later, a camera is placed in front of your neck to see where the iodine is concentrated. People with Hashitoxicosis will have a low RAI uptake result because the thyroid isn't working well and can't absorb much of the RAI. But in people with Graves' disease, the RAI uptake test will be high because the thyroid is absorbing a lot of iodine to produce thyroid hormone.

Although Hashimoto's has no cure, the treatment is fairly simple. You'll need thyroid hormone replacement to replenish your body's missing hormones. Taking replacement hormone will ease the symptoms of hypothyroidism, and in patients who have no symptoms yet, may even prevent hypothyroidism from developing at all.

🩺 Alert

Too much iodine in someone with untreated Hashimoto's can cause enlargement of a goiter. It can also cause a worsening of hypothyroid symptoms. So if you suspect you might have Hashimoto's, steer clear of high-iodine products, which include kelp, seaweed, and certain antiseptics and medicines.

The replacement hormone also halts the excess release of TSH from the pituitary gland, thereby preventing a goiter from developing. In patients who already have a goiter, the drugs can cause the goiter to shrink, though it may take as long as eighteen months.

In some people, the drugs will have no impact on a goiter, and you may need to have your thyroid gland removed. For more information on thyroid hormone replacement, see Chapter 5.

Some doctors may be reluctant to treat you if your TSH levels are normal, despite the presence of autoantibodies that suggest you have Hashimoto's. Other doctors may be willing to start treatment based solely on the presence of autoantibodies. Research suggests that treatment may actually slow the progression of Hashimoto's. A study published in 2001 found that treating people who had normal levels of TSH and autoantibodies for Hashimoto's for a year actually slowed the progression of disease. Upon testing, they found that the people who took levothyroxine had fewer markers for autoimmune disease compared with the patients who did not receive levothyroxine.

Complications

Most people who have Hashimoto's will experience relief once they start taking their thyroid hormone replacement medication. Although it may take some time to establish the proper dosage, you should experience quick relief from your symptoms once you do. But because Hashimoto's is a permanent condition that tends to progress, your TSH levels will need to be monitored regularly. Over time, you may need to adjust the dosage of your medication.

For some people with Hashimoto's, the health problems may go beyond the thyroid to include other autoimmune diseases. That's because autoimmune diseases tend to run in families, and having one condition puts you at risk for others. So if you have Hashimoto's, you are also at increased risk for developing other autoimmune problems.

L. Essential

If you come from a family where autoimmune diseases are rampant or thyroid disorders are common, consider asking your doctor for routine thyroid tests every two years. Catching and treating it early on can help you dodge the bothersome symptoms of Hashimoto's or at least minimize them.

Although the majority of people with Hashimoto's will not develop any other disorders, it's important to know what some of these autoimmune conditions are in case you do start to experience symptoms. Keep in mind, too, that you may be more likely to develop Hashimoto's if you have one of these other conditions.

If you develop multiple autoimmune diseases, the condition is called polyglandular failure syndrome type 2, or Schmidt's syndrome. In polyglandular failure syndrome type 2, the most common endocrine abnormalities are Hashimoto's or Graves' disease, Addison's disease, type 1 diabetes, pernicious anemia, celiac disease, and vitiligo. Polyglandular failure syndrome type 1 only rarely affects the thyroid but does involve frequent fungal infections of the fingers and mouth, low calcium, and Addison's disease.

Type 1 Diabetes

When an autoimmune attack occurs in the insulin-producing beta cells of the pancreas, the result is type 1 diabetes, a condition that often begins in childhood but can also occur in adulthood. Insulin is an essential hormone involved in converting the glucose from food into energy for your body cells to function. People who have type 1 diabetes need to have insulin injections—as do some people who have type 2 diabetes—to replenish the natural hormone that their bodies lack.

Fact

These days, you hear a great deal about the growing incidence of diabetes in the U.S. population. Although the incidence of type 1 diabetes has gone up slightly, the bulk of that increase refers to the rise in type 2 diabetes, which has been fueled by a parallel increase in the numbers of people who are overweight and obese.

Type 1 diabetes that occurs in polyglandular failure syndrome is similar to type 1 diabetes that occurs alone, but it tends to occur in adults. People who have it will notice extreme thirst and frequent urination. You may also experience inexplicable weight loss or flu-like symptoms. As the disease progresses, you may notice blurred vision, numbness and tingling, and cuts and infections that are slow to heal.

Type 1 diabetes is not the same condition as type 2 diabetes, which develops when body cells are no longer sensitive to insulin or when the pancreas doesn't make enough or gradually stops producing insulin. In type 1 diabetes, antibodies are actively attacking the beta cells and destroying their insulin-producing capabilities. Approximately 1 million people in the United States suffer from type 1 diabetes.

Pernicious Anemia

Pernicious anemia, also called megaloblastic anemia, is a rare condition that occurs when the body cannot properly absorb vitamin B12, resulting in a decrease in the production of red blood cells. As a result, you may feel weak and tired. You may also experience an abnormally rapid heartbeat, chest pains, and stomach problems. Some people may also notice a yellowing of the skin, which is called jaundice.

Experts believe that pernicious anemia is an autoimmune condition caused by an attack on a substance in the stomach called intrinsic factor. Most people who have pernicious anemia are lacking in intrinsic factor, which binds to B12 in food and enables its absorption. The condition is more common in older adults, but it may affect younger people who have had problems with anemia in the past. Treatment for pernicious anemia involves getting injections or nasal puffs of B12.

Addison's Disease

Addison's disease occurs when the adrenal glands, which are just above the kidneys, don't produce enough cortisol, the fight-or-flight hormone that prepares your body's reaction to stressful events. Cortisol helps maintain blood pressure and cardiovascular function; slows the immune system's inflammatory response; and aids in the metabolism of carbohydrates, proteins, and fats. Sometimes, the adrenal gland also stops producing enough of a hormone called aldosterone.

Fact

President John F. Kennedy was diagnosed with Addison's disease in 1947. During the presidential race against Lyndon Johnson, the Democrats leaked this information to the media. But the youthful-looking president and his personal physician denied that he had Addison's. In reality, he was on daily cortisone for the rest of his life.

In most cases, Addison's disease is the result of an autoimmune attack on the outer layer of the adrenal glands, which destroys its hormone-producing capabilities. People who have Addison's disease may experience weight loss, fatigue, and weakness. You may also develop low blood pressure and darkening of the skin.

Vitiligo

Vitiligo causes white patches on the skin as the result of an immune attack on the melanocytes, the cells in the skin that give it its color, or pigment. Hair that grows on these discolored patches of skin may sometimes continue to grow, but it, too, will turn white. The condition also affects melanocytes in the mucous membranes of the mouth and nose, the retina of the eye, as well as the rectal and genital areas.

Vitiligo affects 2 to 5 million people in the United States and strikes men and women of all races equally. The disease tends to occur in adults under the age of forty and is more common in people whose parents have the disorder.

Celiac Disease

With celiac disease, eating a protein called gluten, which is found in wheat, rye, barley, and oats, sets off an autoimmune reaction. The ingested gluten triggers a toxic reaction that damages the lining of the small intestine, inhibiting the absorption of vital nutrients. About 2 million people in the United States have celiac disease. The only way to treat the condition is to eat a gluten-free diet.

Alopecia Areata

People with alopecia areata lose their hair when the immune system attacks the hair follicles, causing significant hair loss and balding, often in patches. The condition often begins in childhood and can be psychologically devastating. In the United States, alopecia affects approximately 4.7 million people.

Other Autoimmune Conditions

According to the American Autoimmune Related Diseases Association, there are more than eighty autoimmune conditions.

Autoimmune conditions afflict approximately 20 percent of the U.S. population, or 50 million people. The vast majority are women. Hashimoto's is one of the most common autoimmune conditions, as is Graves' disease.

The severity of these conditions varies widely among individuals. Some conditions may be mild and produce virtually no symptoms. Others may require intensive treatment and can be life-threatening. Becoming familiar with these diseases is important to someone with Hashimoto's since your risk for these diseases is now statistically higher than someone who does not have Hashimoto's. The following are some other autoimmune conditions you might hear about.

Systemic Lupus Erythematosus (SLE)

SLE occurs when the body's immune system attacks connective tissue, and can affect virtually every part of the body, but especially the skin, joints, blood, and kidneys. People with lupus frequently have achy joints, a low-grade fever, a butterfly rash on the face, and extreme fatigue. Experts estimate there are 500,000 to 1.5 million Americans who have been diagnosed with lupus.

Rheumatoid arthritis

Rheumatoid arthritis occurs when the immune system attacks the lining of the joints, causing swelling, warmth, and pain. The condition can be extremely painful, difficult to treat, and in some cases, debilitating. Some people experience deformities around the joints. The condition afflicts about 2.1 million people, the majority of them women.

Sjogren's Syndrome

People who have Sjogren's syndrome lose the ability to produce tears and saliva as the result of an autoimmune attack on the body's moisture-producing glands. The dryness can also affect other organs such as the lungs, kidneys, and gastrointestinal tract. The condition affects 4 million people, mostly women, and commonly occurs with other autoimmune diseases.

Inflammatory Bowel Disease

Inflammatory bowel disease actually refers to a family of conditions, the two most common being Crohn's disease and ulcerative colitis. Crohn's disease is the inflammation of the GI tract, usually the small intestine. Ulcerative colitis affects the top layer of the colon. Symptoms include diarrhea, cramps, fever, and sometimes bleeding. Together, these conditions affect about a million people.

Essential

Most autoimmune conditions will wax and wane between periods of remission and flare-ups. While it's hard to pinpoint what exactly causes the disease to flare, one factor that seems to be involved is stress. If you do have an autoimmune condition—or any chronic condition for that matter—take steps to minimize your stress.

Multiple Sclerosis (MS)

MS is the autoimmune destruction of the myelin sheath, or covering, of the nerves. This condition can affect the entire central nervous system, causing muscle weakness, poor balance, spasticity, numbness, pain, and vision problems. The condition affects 200,000 to 350,000 people in the United States.

Others Forms of Thyroiditis

Hashimoto's disease is the most common cause of thyroiditis, but there are other conditions that can cause your thyroid gland to become inflamed. Some of these are fairly common, and others are really rather rare. Still, if your thyroid gland is inflamed and blood tests have ruled out Hashimoto's, it's quite possible that you have another form of thyroiditis.

Subacute Thyroiditis

You arrive at the doctor's office complaining of a sore throat and flulike symptoms. Moments later, after touching your neck, your doctor says that the real culprit may be a thyroid problem. Chances are, you have subacute thyroiditis, which is sometimes called deQuervain's thyroiditis, named for the Swiss surgeon who first described the condition in 1904.

Subacute thyroiditis usually occurs after a bout of the flu or another upper respiratory infection. It has also been linked to other viral diseases, including mumps and Coxsackie virus. Usually, patients will notice pain in the lower neck and rapid enlargement of the thyroid gland. Some people may develop a fever, hoarseness, and difficulty swallowing. In some cases, the condition is mild and barely noticeable and simply goes away on its own.

For other people, however, the condition may be more progressive. During the early stages, as the thyroid gland releases excess hormone into the bloodstream, subacute thyroiditis may cause symptoms of hyperthyroidism, such as nervousness, anxiety, a rapid heartbeat, and an intolerance for heat. After a while, these symptoms will evolve into those of hypothyroidism, with fatigue, forgetfulness, dry skin, and intolerance for the cold becoming more prominent.

Diagnosing subacute thyroiditis can be tricky and is often a process of elimination. The most obvious sign is a painful neck. But other indicators in the blood, such as the erythrocyte sedimentation rate, may also reveal a great deal of inflammation. If necessary, an RAI uptake test might be done. Results that are low would reveal very little uptake of iodine in the inflamed thyroid.

Treatment for subacute thyroiditis usually involves bed rest and aspirin to reduce the inflammation. In more severe cases, cortisone may be given to tame the inflammation, and thyroid hormone replacement may be needed to restore the missing hormones. But the condition usually resolves itself after several weeks or months, and the thyroid gland returns to normal function. In rare cases, you may be placed on thyroid hormone for good if normal thyroid function does not resume.

Fact

Inflammation in the body can be detected by measuring erythrocyte sedimentation rate, or sed rate. The test measures how quickly red blood cells settle in a test tube. When there is inflammation, certain proteins called erythrocytes will settle faster and result in a higher sed rate.

Silent Thyroiditis

Silent thyroiditis is just that: a quiet condition that produces no obvious symptoms and causes no pain. And yet, the thyroid is inflamed. The only way to know you have it is if you develop symptoms of hyperthyroidism.

Like subacute thyroiditis, the initial inflammation sometimes causes too much thyroid hormone to leak into the bloodstream, producing symptoms of hyperthyroidism. After a while, you may notice some symptoms of hypothyroidism, as the hormone release slows and the thyroid gland remains inflamed.

The cause of silent thyroiditis is unknown, but tests have found that the thyroid gland in silent thyroiditis is filled with lymphocytes, a type of white blood cell involved in the immune system. For that reason, experts believe that silent thyroiditis is a temporary malfunction of the immune system.

Like the subacute form, silent thyroiditis usually resolves on its own with bed rest and aspirin to treat the inflammation. Usually, no other treatment is needed unless a patient becomes permanently hypothyroid, which is rare.

Postpartum Thyroiditis

Most cases of silent thyroiditis occur after a woman delivers a baby, hence the name *postpartum thyroiditis*. The condition typically occurs four to twelve months after delivery, and is most common in women who already have an autoimmune problem or thyroid disorder. Often, it goes undetected because the woman assumes her symptoms are part of the rigors of new motherhood.

Like silent thyroiditis, the postpartum version follows a similar course of events: inflammation of the gland leads first to symptoms of hyperthyroidism, followed by a period of hypothyroidism.

Alert

It's easy to confuse hypothyroidism caused by postpartum thyroiditis with postpartum depression. The two conditions share several of the same symptoms, including depression, fatigue, and mood swings. But the two are distinct conditions. If your sadness persists, seek professional help. Postpartum depression is a serious disorder that can endanger both the mother and the baby.

In some cases of postpartum thyroiditis, there is no treatment, just the passage of time. The condition usually resolves itself twelve to eighteen months after it starts. But if symptoms are more severe, you may be given an antithyroid drug such as propylthiouracil (PTU) or beta-blockers, which slow your heart rate, for hyperthyroidism, or thyroid hormone replacement for hypothyroidism. You will still be able to breast-feed while taking these medications.

Acute Suppurative Thyroiditis

In rare cases, bacteria can invade the thyroid gland, particularly the left lobe, and trigger inflammation. Acute suppurative thyroiditis is a bacterial infection of the thyroid that is extremely rare and tends to occur in children. The infection causes pus to form and the thyroid gland to become extremely painful. The condition also causes fever and chills as the body battles the infection.

Acute thyroiditis is treated with antibiotics. In more severe cases, you may need surgery to drain the infection. But the condition generally does not cause any long-term problems with the thyroid.

Riedel's Thyroiditis

Riedel's thyroiditis is an extremely rare condition that involves the buildup of scar tissue in and around the thyroid gland. In Riedel's, the thyroid gland becomes inflamed and attaches itself to nearby tissues such as the windpipe (trachea) or your vocal cords. The growth of fibrous tissue is painless but may make it hard to swallow. You may also notice that your voice is deeper than normal, and that you have some trouble breathing. Eventually, the thyroid gland becomes very hard and enlarged.

Usually, you will need a biopsy to determine whether it is inflammation or cancer that is causing the thyroid to harden and enlarge. Treatment depends on the extent of the disease, and may range from the use of steroids to surgery. If the condition destroys the hormone-production capability of the thyroid gland, you will need replacement hormone.

CHAPTER 7

Hyperthyroidism

You're nervous, edgy, and your heart feels as if it's always racing. At night, you can't sleep. During the day, you feel warm and sweaty. If your thyroid is the culprit, you may have hyperthyroidism, which does exactly what the name suggests: It makes you hyper. Calming the overactive thyroid requires action to slow everything down. Read on to learn more about this once deadly disease. This chapter covers the details of hyperthyroidism—from diagnosis to treatment.

What Is Hyperthyroidism?

Hyperthyroidism occurs when you have an overactive thyroid gland. The result of this excess activity is called thyrotoxicosis, which means that you have too much thyroid hormone circulating in your blood.

Hyperthyroidism is much less common than hypothyroidism. According to the AACE, the condition occurs in almost 1 percent of the U.S. population. Women are affected five to ten times more often than men are.

The cause of hyperthyroidism varies among patients, but identifying the cause is essential to figuring out your treatment. The most common culprit is Graves' disease, an autoimmune condition that we'll discuss in greater detail in another chapter. In Graves' disease, autoantibodies attack the thyroid gland, causing it to release excess amounts of thyroid hormone.

Some people develop hyperthyroidism as the result of toxic multinodular goiter. This condition is most common in adults over the age of sixty, who have been living with an undetected goiter for a long time. In that time, the goiter develops nodules that begin to churn out a supply of thyroid hormone on their own, without any prodding from the pituitary gland.

⌐ Essential

Many patients who have hyperthyroidism develop hypothyroidism after treatment. In some cases, the diseased gland is destroyed intentionally, knowing that the patient will go into a hypothyroid state. But remember, hypothyroidism is easily treated with thyroid replacement hormone. It's much better to be hypothyroid than hyperthyroid.

Hyperthyroidism may also be the result of a single toxic nodule, a condition called Plummer's disease, which was named after Henry Stanley Plummer, an American doctor. Another name for this condition is single hot nodule, or toxic adenoma. Like toxic multinodular goiter, this single nodule will produce more thyroid hormone than your body needs, causing you to become hyperthyroid.

Some people may develop hyperthyroidism as a result of subacute thyroiditis, in which the thyroid gland becomes enlarged, inflamed, and painful. The result of this enlargement is the release of too much thyroid hormone.

In other cases, the hyperthyroidism is the result of silent thyroiditis, in which the thyroid gland becomes painlessly inflamed. After giving birth, about 5 to 10 percent of women may develop a form of this condition called postpartum thyroiditis. In both silent and postpartum thyroiditis, the thyroid may remain overactive for one to two months, followed by several months of hypothyroidism. Eventually, normal thyroid function resumes, though some people become permanently hypothyroid.

Some cases of hyperthyroidism result from eating too much iodine, the mineral the thyroid uses to produce thyroid hormone.

Experts call this iodine-induced hyperthyroidism. It may occur in people who take certain medications such as amiodarone, which is used to treat abnormal heart rhythms. It may also occur in people who take kelp, a type of seaweed that has been touted as a health supplement for numerous ailments.

Finally, some people can develop hyperthyroidism when they are being treated for hypothyroidism. This type of hyperthyroidism may occur when the dose of thyroid hormone replacement is too high. It is usually corrected once the dosage is properly adjusted.

Question

Who is at risk for hyperthyroidism?
Being a woman increases your odds for hyperthyroidism—especially if you're pregnant. The condition is also more common in people between the ages of thirty and fifty. In addition, your risk goes up if you have a family or personal history of thyroid problems. People who have an autoimmune disease such as lupus, rheumatoid arthritis, or type 1 diabetes are more likely to get Graves' disease, a type of hyperthyroidism, as well.

What Hyperthyroidism Looks Like

When your body produces too much thyroid hormone, everything speeds up. In fact, your metabolism may increase by as much as 60 to 100 percent—as much as double its normal speed. As you might imagine, this can produce profound effects on how your body functions and on how you feel.

But as with hypothyroidism, these symptoms may develop slowly. When you first become hyperthyroid, you may feel fine and have no symptoms at all. But gradually, as your thyroid gland becomes increasingly active, you will start to notice changes that will become more bothersome over time.

🩺 Alert

In healthy people, it's normal for your heart to speed up during exercise, activity, or stress. But in people with hyperthyroidism, your heart may beat this fast even when you are sitting still or asleep. If your heart rate goes above 100 beats per minute, you are said to have tachycardia. A sustained rapid heart rate always warrants medical attention.

Your Heart

Most people with hyperthyroidism will notice that their heart is beating faster, even during periods of rest. In some people, the heart rate speeds up to more than 100 beats a minute. In older people, a sped-up heart can lead to irregular rhythms, which can be dangerous in people with other forms of heart disease.

The effects on your heart can be easily measured. Your blood pressure will be higher than normal. Your pulse will be considerably faster. In some people, a sped-up heart can feel as if it is beating out of their chest. The increase in your heart rate can cause other symptoms, too, such as headaches, breathlessness, and dizziness.

Nervousness and Irritability

People with an overactive thyroid frequently feel on edge, nervous, and anxious. They may have trouble catching their breath. They may fidget and experience tremors in their hands. In their dealings with other people, they may be irritable and argumentative. The nervousness often causes difficulties with sleep, leading to frequent bouts of insomnia. Doug says he remembers feeling very agitated.

All his life, Doug always felt as if he had energy to burn. But at thirty-nine, his energy levels seemed to spike. He was quickly agitated, and noticed that he was sweating more than usual while playing basketball. He also started having occasional heart palpitations and wondered if he was having a panic attack. Looking back, he remembers many times when he felt as if he was on a caffeine buzz. Now he wonders if it was his overactive thyroid.

Weight Changes

Many people with hyperthyroidism experience weight loss and changes in their appetite. These changes in weight and appetite are the result of a revved up metabolism that causes your body to burn up energy more rapidly.

Most people notice an increase in their appetite as their body's energy needs increase. But even with the extra food they're eating, many of them may still be losing weight. Other symptoms of hyperthyroidism, including diarrhea and heavy sweating, can compound your weight loss, too.

Still others with hyperthyroidism will lose all interest in eating and rapidly lose weight. If this occurs in teenagers, they may be mistakenly diagnosed with an eating disorder.

Less common, some people's appetites surpass their stepped up metabolic rates, resulting in weight gain. An increase in weight may also be caused in part by extreme exhaustion, which can make it hard for you to exercise or stay active.

The GI Tract

Hyperthyroidism causes your gastrointestinal tract to digest foods more quickly. The excess hormone causes an increase in the contractions in your bowels. As a result, you may notice more frequent bowel movements or, in more severe cases, diarrhea.

The Eyes

The eyes are sensitive to the effects of thyroid hormone, and patients with severe hyperthyroidism will develop a stare in which the eyes appear to have a wide-eyed, startled appearance.

This condition is common in people who have Graves' disease and is called thyroid eye disease, or infiltrative ophthalmology. With thyroid eye disease, the eyeball bulges. This bulging is caused by swelling in the muscles around the eyes, which makes the eyeball protrude. Some hyperthyroid patients may have trouble closing their eyes completely. With the eyeball constantly exposed, the eye can become red and irritated.

L. Essential

Early on, irritations of the eye may be mild and mistaken for allergies, especially since many of the symptoms are most noticeable in air-conditioning, hot-air heating, and windy climates. You may also have trouble wearing contact lenses because they are irritating. If these symptoms occur with other symptoms, ask your doctor to consider your thyroid.

In more severe cases, the eyes lose the ability to move in sync, and you may experience double vision. Many people may also notice that their eyes are more sensitive to light, and that they frequently feel gritty, dry, and irritated.

Enlarged Thyroid Gland

An overactive thyroid causes your thyroid gland to develop a goiter, which means the gland has become enlarged. If you put your hand on the goiter, you may notice a vibration called a thrill, caused by an increase in blood flow to the thyroid.

Emotional Disturbances

Hyperthyroidism can lead to a host of emotional disturbances that produce symptoms of depression and mania. In extreme cases, it can cause disordered thinking or delusional thoughts. Some people may actually receive a psychiatric misdiagnosis for these extreme mood swings.

Many of the emotional problems come from the sheer exhaustion that results from having hyperthyroidism. The body becomes exhausted by the increased energy burn, which is made worse by lack of sleep.

Other Changes

People who have hyperthyroidism are often intolerant of the heat and may sweat profusely in temperatures that healthy people consider comfortable. Their skin may feel moist to the touch. They may also notice muscle weakness, especially in the thighs and the upper arms or shoulders. In addition, they may bruise more easily, lose hair, and experience frequent, loose stools.

Hyperthyroidism frequently causes changes in your hair, skin, and nails. Many people notice a thinning of the skin. The excess perspiration may cause a rash. Hair may become finer and softer, and you may also notice hair loss on your scalp. Fingernails may grow more rapidly and separate from the nail bed.

Women with hyperthyroidism may notice their periods are lighter and may even skip periods. Men may experience erectile dysfunction. Both men and women may notice a drop in libido. Because of these effects on sexual function, hyperthyroidism can cause fertility problems for couples trying to conceive.

Alert

If you don't have your menstrual period for three months or more, call your doctor. Amenorrhea—the absence of regular periods—may also be caused by polycystic ovarian syndrome or Cushing's disease, an overproduction of the hormone cortisol. Women who exercise in excess or who are under extreme stress also may stop menstruating.

Left untreated, hyperthyroidism can lead to serious consequences. Excess thyroid hormone can make it hard for your bones to take up calcium, which can lead to osteoporosis. The impact on your heart can lead to heart failure, which occurs when your heart can't pump enough blood to the organs, resulting in death. You can also develop dangerous arrhythmias.

Making the Diagnosis

In most cases, a thorough physical exam and a simple blood test are all it takes to determine whether you're suffering from hyperthyroidism.

The more challenging aspect of a diagnosis is figuring out the type of hyperthyroidism you have, which is critical to determining your treatment. A comprehensive diagnosis then involves several components.

Before any blood is drawn, your doctor should engage you in a conversation about your health. Some signs of hyperthyroidism are easily measured or observed by a physician, such as your pulse or bulging eyes. But it's up to you to tell your doctor about the symptoms—those he can't see or measure—that you are suffering.

Perhaps you're perspiring more than usual. Or maybe your once-wavy hair can no longer hold a curl. Maybe you're having trouble sleeping and are feeling anxious. All these are symptoms of hyperthyroidism. The information you provide is critical to helping him weed out other disorders, such as generalized anxiety disorder and low blood sugar.

Keep in mind, too, that a history of hyperthyroidism increases the odds that you'll have it again. Candace, for example, had a recurrence ten years after her first episode.

Her first bout was the result of subacute thyroiditis after a viral infection. She shed thirty pounds in a month and had severe pain in her neck, a racing heart, tremors, and anxiety. After several months on beta-blockers, the condition disappeared, and Candace was fine for ten years. Then she had poison ivy and developed hives. She began to lose weight again, and felt anxious and had trouble concentrating. Although she initially blamed her symptoms on stress, a visit to her doctor told her otherwise—Candace had hyperthyroidism again.

Blood Tests

One of the most important things your doctor will do is order blood tests to figure out if you have hyperthyroidism. Blood tests are critical in determining whether your thyroid is causing your bothersome symptoms. It's a relatively simple process, but interpreting the results can be tricky.

TSH

Like hypothyroidism, hyperthyroidism can be measured with a simple test to determine your TSH levels. The TSH test is considered by most doctors to be the single best screening tool for hyperthyroidism.

Fact

Some groups recommend regular screening for thyroid disease. The American Thyroid Association (ATA) for instance, recommends that adults older than thirty-five be screened with a TSH test every five years. The TSH is used to detect both hyper- and hypothyroidism. But the U.S. Preventive Services Task Force recommends against any routine screening. Some groups suggest screening women before and after pregnancy, whereas others recommend screening adults over age fifty or sixty.

As you might recall, TSH is the hormone secreted by the pituitary gland that tells the thyroid gland to release more T4. The American College of Clinical Endocrinologists currently considers normal levels of TSH to be in the range of 0.3 to 3.0 mIU/dL. When your body produces enough thyroid hormone, your TSH levels stabilize in the normal range. But when your body has too much thyroid hormone, it automatically shuts down the release of TSH.

Sometimes, a TSH test is not enough. TSH levels may be low in both hyperthyroidism and hypothyroidism due to a pituitary disorder (central hypopituitarism, see Chapter 12). In that case, other tests are needed to help your doctor determine if you have hyperthyroidism.

Total T3 and Free T3

When it comes to diagnosing hyperthyroidism, levels of total T3 are generally an accurate tool. Total T3 reveals the amount of the active form of thyroid hormone, both the form that binds to proteins and the form that gets into body cells. Too much of it indicates that you have an overactive thyroid. In some patients, especially the elderly, the test can reveal T3 toxicosis, a condition in which too much T3, but normal amounts of T4, is being released from the thyroid and causing hyperthyroid symptoms.

Although knowing your total T3, along with your TSH, is often enough to determine whether you have hyperthyroidism, a free T3 test is sometimes taken, especially if your free T4 results are normal and you're still having symptoms of hyperthyroidism.

Total T4 and Free T4

Total T4 is a measure of all the T4 in your body, including the T4 that is bound to protein and unavailable to body cells for use. Since the bulk of the T4 released by your thyroid is bound to proteins, it is usually a less than accurate measure of hyperthyroidism. Abnormal levels of total T4 may reveal problems with protein binding and not thyroid problems. Still, it may be one more clue that you have hyperthyroidism, and your doctor may request it as an additional piece of information.

A more reliable measure is free T4. This test measures the remaining T4, or free thyroxine, in the blood. Free T4 is the thyroid hormone available to enter body cells, where it can be converted into T3, the active part of thyroid hormone. In patients who have hyperthyroidism, free T4 levels can be higher than normal.

Thyroid Autoantibodies

When viruses or bacteria invade your body, the immune system releases antibodies that attack the invaders. But in people who have an autoimmune condition, the body mistakenly attacks healthy tissue with destructive autoantibodies. When the thyroid gland suffers an autoimmune attack, the body produces several antibodies. Lab tests to detect these substances offer further evidence that your thyroid disease is the result of an autoimmune reaction.

Essential

Some people who have other autoimmune diseases such as rheumatoid arthritis, Sjogren's syndrome, lupus, and pernicious anemia may also have thyroid-stimulating immunoglobulin (TSI) antibodies in their blood. The odds of having these antibodies increase with age, and they are more common in women.

Testing for TSI can be done to determine if the hyperthyroidism is caused by Graves' disease. In healthy people, TSH from the pituitary gland will bind to TSH receptors on the thyroid cell, triggering it to produce thyroid hormone. In people with Graves' disease, TSI will take over the action of TSH, bind to the TSH receptor, and trigger the release of T4 and T3. But when thyroid hormone levels become too high, TSI, unlike TSH, doesn't stop stimulating the production of thyroid hormone, causing levels to soar to unhealthy heights.

Radioactive Iodine Uptake (RAIU) and Scan

Diagnosing and treating hyperthyroidism requires more than just knowing whether your thyroid gland is overactive. You also need to know what's causing it to act up. That's why you'll need these other tests to identify the cause behind your hyperthyroidism.

The RAIU and scan, critical tests that are usually done together, measure how much iodine the thyroid gland collects and can help your doctor determine whether your overactive thyroid is the result of Graves' disease, toxic multinodular goiter, or thyroiditis.

Your doctor may suggest fasting for eight hours before the test in order to reduce the amount of iodine in your body. You should also alert your doctor to any medications and supplements you take, since many of these substances may contain iodine and can affect the results of the test.

Question

Is radioactive iodine safe?
Many people get nervous when they hear the term radioactive. But the form of radioactive iodine used in radioactive iodine uptake (RAIU) is highly safe. The dose is very low. Pregnant and nursing women, however, should not undergo an RAIU since the radioactive iodine does cross the placenta, is passed in breast milk, and can affect the baby.

The RAIU test is usually done in the nuclear medicine department of a hospital. The test involves ingesting a pill or liquid that contains small amounts of radioactive iodine-123. After six to twenty-four hours—and sometimes at several intervals—you will return for a measurement of the radioactivity (uptake) and a picture of your thyroid (scan). The scan will reveal where the iodine is concentrated in the thyroid gland. The scan also reveals which parts of the gland are functioning normally by taking up iodine, and which parts are not.

Here's what your doctor might find:

- If the hyperthyroidism is caused by Graves' disease, the uptake and scan will show the thyroid is red or "hot," indicating higher than normal amounts of iodine in the thyroid gland. The scan will show diffuse uptake of the iodine over the whole thyroid.

- If the cause is subacute thyroiditis, the uptake will be low because the excess hormone is coming from stored thyroid hormone and not being made in the thyroid gland.
- If the cause is toxic multinodular goiter, the thyroid will appear patchy, with the nodules that are producing excess hormone showing up hot and the rest of the thyroid appearing cold. The overall uptake is elevated but less so than in Graves' disease.
- If the cause is a single nodule, the scan and uptake will be hot only where the nodule is located.
- If the cause is too much thyroid hormone replacement, the scan and uptake will appear cold since the hormone is coming from medication and not the thyroid itself.

In some cases, the patient is injected with an RAI isotope. Again, you'll be asked to return after six to twenty-four hours—and sometimes at several different intervals—and asked to lie on a table, with your head stretched back, so that the neck is exposed. A camera is then used to scan your neck for radiation.

Fact

In addition to blood work and the RAIU test and scan, your doctor may also order other types of tests to help make a diagnosis. For instance, a computerized tomography (CT) scan may be used to detect a goiter or large nodules. An ultrasound may be performed to find out whether the thyroid is enlarged. Once you're receiving treatment for hyperthyroidism, your doctor may do an ultrasound of the thyroid to see if your thyroid has gotten smaller.

Doing a thyroid scan can help your doctor figure out which parts of the gland are functioning normally and which parts are not. An overactive gland will take up more than normal amounts of iodine, while an underactive gland will take up less. A scan can also reveal the presence of one or more overactive nodules, which will take up more than normal amounts of iodine. In addition, a scan can reveal the presence of a tumor, which would appear cold.

An RAIU test and scan is critical to identifying the cause of your hyperthyroidism. Combined with a physical exam and a discussion of your symptoms, the test can help lead you to the best treatment, too.

Putting It Together

Figuring out that you have hyperthyroidism isn't always easy. Pinpointing the cause is even tougher. Lower than normal levels of TSH generally suggest an overactive thyroid, but your doctor may need other tests as well as your self-reported symptoms before reaching a conclusive diagnosis.

In some people, the tests may all come back normal, despite the presence of bothersome symptoms. If that happens to you, make sure to request follow-up testing in six months. But if the tests are not normal, you will probably be given a diagnosis of some form of hyperthyroidism.

Mild (Subclinical) Hyperthyroidism

If your TSH levels are lower than normal but your free T4 and free T3 tests are normal or slightly high, you are said to have mild or subclinical hyperthyroidism. Experts don't always agree on whether you need treatment at this point, but routine monitoring and evaluations are important regardless.

Detecting subclinical hyperthyroidism is especially difficult. The only clue might be a slightly lower than normal TSH level. Nonetheless, treatment can be important, especially in older patients, who are at greater risk for heart problems and osteoporosis.

Hyperthyroidism

If your TSH level is low or nonexistent and your free T4 and T3 levels are normal to high, you will probably be diagnosed with basic hyperthyroidism.

Graves' Disease

If you test positive for TSI antibodies and have a low or nonexistent TSH level and normal to high free T4 and T3 levels, you may be diagnosed with Graves' disease. Your scan will show increased radioactivity throughout the gland. You may also have TPO antibodies, but because TPO also occurs in Hashimoto's disease, your doctor will need to make sure to perform the TSI antibodies test to ensure an accurate diagnosis.

Pituitary Hyperthyroidism

Rarely, tumors on the pituitary gland called adenomas may secrete TSH, causing the thyroid to produce too much thyroid hormone. In this case, your TSH is high, and your free T4 and free T3 tend to be elevated.

Challenges in Diagnosis

Hyperthyroidism isn't easy to diagnose because many symptoms mimic those of other conditions. Patients may complain about individual symptoms such as insomnia, tremors, or nervousness, and doctors may simply treat these bothersome symptoms with a sleep remedy or antidepressant while ignoring the bigger picture.

In some cases, the hyperthyroid patient is misdiagnosed as having a psychiatric illness. That's because many of the symptoms of hyperthyroidism affect emotions and behavior. People who have an overactive thyroid are often jittery, nervous, and anxious. They may have what they believe are panic attacks. They may be easily provoked, and in rare cases, may have bizarre or delusional thought patterns.

⌐ Essential

A panic attack can feel like an intense episode of stress, but it occurs without any obvious provocation or warning. Generally, each attack lasts just a few minutes. According to the American Psychological Association, the key symptom in panic disorder is your fear of having future attacks. Patients with panic disorder will have normal thyroid tests.

To make matters worse, many people with hyperthyroidism have trouble sleeping. The fatigue only worsens the exhaustion and emotional difficulties, making you even more irritable, jittery, and anxious. If you notice that you are suffering from these kinds of symptoms, consider your thyroid a possible culprit. A simple blood test is all it takes to diagnose or rule out a thyroid problem.

The Importance of Treatment

Untreated hyperthyroidism can cause serious complications, even death. Left unchecked, the condition can also weaken bones and cause damage to the eyes that results in double vision, blurring, and sensitivity to light. And if you are a woman who plans to have children, it can raise your risk for birth defects and miscarriages. Fortunately, proper treatment will reduce your risks. But you should still be aware of the potential for certain medical problems.

Heart Disease

Almost everyone who has hyperthyroidism experiences tachycardia, in which the heart beat becomes rapid and beats more than 100 times a minute. Some people may describe these as palpitations. Palpitations are sometimes a sign of an arrhythmia, in which the heartbeat has become irregular.

In addition, some people may develop an abnormal heart rhythm called an atrial fibrillation. With atrial fibrillations, the heart will have random pauses interspersed with bursts of rapid heartbeats. The condition is most likely to occur in hyperthyroid patients who have an underlying heart condition. Left untreated, atrial fibrillations can cause blood clots that lead to stroke.

 Fact

Heart disease is the leading cause of death in both men and women in the United States. According to the Centers for Disease Control and Prevention, studies have shown that making lifestyle changes to lower high cholesterol and high blood pressure can reduce your risk for dying of heart disease, having a fatal heart attack, and needing bypass surgery. For information on how, check out the American Heart Association Web site at *www.americanheart.org*.

Some hyperthyroid patients experience what is called high output failure. In this case, the heart is pumping so fast that it doesn't have time to fill up with blood. As a result, the heart becomes incapable of pumping enough blood to the body's organs, causing swelling and shortness of breath. Over time, the heart is forced to work harder and harder, eventually causing death. Here are some other problems that can occur with hyperthyroidism:

- **Angina:** Angina describes the chest pain or squeezing sensation that occurs when the heart can't get enough oxygen as the result of plaque buildup in artery walls.
- **Heart Attack:** Also known as a myocardial infarction, a heart attack occurs when a coronary artery to the heart is blocked off by a blood clot, causing damage or death to the heart muscle.
- **Heart Failure:** Previously known as congestive heart failure, heart failure occurs when the heart can't pump enough

blood to meet the body's needs, causing fatigue, shortness of breath, and fluid buildup in lungs and body tissue.

In otherwise healthy people who develop hyperthyroidism, arrhythmias and tachycardia are usually temporary conditions. But if you have other risk factors for heart disease, such as high blood pressure, high cholesterol, and obesity, hyperthyroidism can be dangerous and raise your risk for heart problems. Prompt treatment can lessen your risk, and serious heart problems can usually be averted once the hyperthyroidism is treated.

Bone Loss

Our bones are in a constant state of flux. Osteoblasts build new bone, while osteoclasts break down old bone. When you develop hyperthyroidism, these osteoclasts go into overdrive and break down bone at a rapid rate. But the osteoblasts are not affected by the excess thyroid hormone, and so they can't keep up with the destruction. The result is bone loss, and in the extreme, osteoporosis, a condition in which the bones are severely weakened.

Unless you suffer a fracture, however, you probably won't even know you have osteoporosis. The condition is painless and produces no symptoms. But if you have osteoporosis and you fall, the conditioning can become life-threatening. Bone loss is especially problematic in older, postmenopausal women, who may already have weakened bones.

Thyroid Storm

In some people, if hyperthyroidism is severe, a condition called thyroid storm may develop. Thyroid storm produces intense and severe symptoms of hyperthyroidism, primarily affecting the heart. Fortunately, the incidence of thyroid storm has gone down significantly with earlier and better treatments. That's why getting properly diagnosed and treated for hyperthyroidism is so important. In the next chapter, we'll examine your treatment options.

CHAPTER 8

Treating Hyperthyroidism

Now that you know you have hyperthyroidism, it's essential to get properly treated—and promptly. Not only are the symptoms of hyperthyroidism extremely bothersome, but left untreated, the condition could eventually cause heart problems and bone loss. In this chapter, you'll find an outline of your treatment options—from RAI to antithyroid drugs. Once you've become educated about all the choices, you can work with your doctor to pin down the option that works best for you.

Treatment Options

Unlike the treatment for hypothyroidism, which is fairly straightforward and involves thyroid hormone replacement, getting relief from hyperthyroidism can be more complicated. Deciding on a course of treatment depends on the type of hyperthyroidism you have, the severity of your condition, and how well you respond to other treatments.

Many people are treated with RAI to ablate—or destroy—the thyroid tissue that is making too much hormone. Others are given antithyroid medications that slow the production of thyroid hormone. In rare cases, hyperthyroidism is treated with surgery to remove the parts of your thyroid that are producing the excess hormone. In addition to taming the overactive thyroid gland itself, you may need treatments for the effects of the disease, such as the rapid heart rate and the eye problems.

Knowing as much as you can about each form of treatment will help you work with your doctor on choosing the best way to handle your overactive thyroid.

Radioactive Iodine (RAI)

RAI treatment works by destroying some or all of the thyroid tissue that is producing too much thyroid hormone. RAI is the only way to ablate parts of the thyroid gland without causing harm to other parts of the body. The technique relies on the fact that the thyroid gland is the only part of the body that takes up iodine.

Before RAI treatment, you will have an RAIU scan to confirm that you have hyperthyroidism and that the cause is not thyroiditis, which does not respond to RAI. Unlike the diagnostic scans, RAI uses a stronger radioactive isotope, namely iodine-131, instead of iodine-123. In patients who take up low levels of the RAI, a medication called Thyrogen may be used. Thyrogen is a synthetic version of TSH that has the same effect on thyroid cells—it encourages them to take up the RAI.

Alert

RAI treatment should never be used in women who are pregnant or nursing. And women who are trying to conceive should wait at least six months to a year after RAI before even trying to get pregnant.

The actual treatment is fairly simple. Beforehand, you may be asked to eat a low-iodine diet for a few weeks to ensure that other sources of iodine do not interfere with the RAI. The treatment is then given orally by pill or liquid in the nuclear medicine division of a hospital. The substance travels into the bloodstream, where it is picked up by the overactive disease cells in the thyroid. Once there, the RAI destroys the diseased thyroid tissue.

Precautions to Take

After treatment, though the amount of radioactivity is small, you may be advised to take precautions for the first week or two, so that your radioactivity does not contaminate others. The RAI is eventually excreted in the urine, and also in saliva and sweat. Here are some precautions to follow:

- Drink a lot of water. The fluid will help flush the RAI from your body.
- Avoid intimate contact with others, such as kissing and hugging, especially with small children and pregnant women.
- Wash all glasses, utensils, and dishes immediately after use.
- Flush toilets two or three times after each use.
- Separate your clothes, linens, and towels from others'.
- Sleep alone.
- Avoid preparing food for others, if possible. If you must, wash your hands carefully beforehand.
- Maintain a reasonable physical distance from other people.

Also, if you travel by plane shortly after RAI treatment, carry a letter from your doctor explaining your recent therapy. Some detection devices can be triggered by even the slightest amount of radiation.

Although highly effective, it will probably take a few months to know for sure whether the RAI has succeeded and for your symptoms to fade completely. During that time, you will undergo routine tests to measure the amounts of thyroid hormone in your blood.

In most people, RAI is highly successful and safe. The procedure, which has been in use since the 1950s, does not increase your risk for thyroid cancer, although most people become hypothyroid afterward.

Sometimes, finding the perfect dose of RAI can be very difficult. High doses of RAI are more likely to be successful, but almost guarantee that you'll be hypothyroid in the end. A lower, more conservative amount of RAI often doesn't work. Too little treatment, and you wind up still battling hyperthyroidism. In some cases, the RAI may make you euthyroid—meaning you have normal thyroid levels—for a year or so, before you develop hyperthyroidism again or hypothy-roidism after that.

L. Essential

> People who have severe thyroid eye disease caused by Graves' dis-ease may not be good candidates for RAI. The treatments tend to cause a worsening of the eye symptoms. But if RAI is necessary, you may want to consider taking steroids, which seem to lessen the effects on the eyes.

For most people, a single treatment is sometimes all it takes to be cured of hyperthyroidism. About a third of all patients will need a second dose. And in rare cases, a third dose may become necessary. These numbers depend on the dose of RAI used.

Side Effects

After treatment, you may notice some pain or tenderness in the neck, which can be treated with over-the-counter pain remedies. Some people may experience nausea or vomiting, especially if they've received a higher dose. You may notice some dryness in the mouth and a decrease in the production of saliva. Eating sour can-dies, lemons, or pickles can sometimes stimulate the salivary glands and eliminate the dryness.

In some cases, patients may experience an increase in their symptoms of hyperthyroidism. This development is caused by the death of the diseased cells, which are spilling thyroid hormone into the bloodstream. This side effect is more problematic in older adults, who may have heart problems as a result. Treatment with antithy-roid drugs or other medications can usually relieve the symptoms. Fortunately, this is typically a temporary situation that disappears as the cells die off for good.

Fact

Former Olympic gold medalist Gail Devers had RAI treatments for her hyperthyroidism from Graves' disease. Before winning the gold medal in the 100-meter dash in 1992, Devers's condition was so severe that doctors had considered amputating her feet, which had become blistered and swollen. Fortunately, a correct diagnosis was made in time for treatment—and future Olympic success. She won gold again in the same event in 1996.

Some people may experience temporary bouts of hypothyroidism in the six months after RAI treatment and then become euthyroid. But many people who undergo RAI become permanently hypothyroid. In fact, research suggests that as many as 50 percent of all people who undergo RAI will develop hypothyroidism. The risk rises with each successive treatment. That's why it's important to get routine thyroid function tests if you've received RAI. Joan, for example, recalls the pendulum of being first hyperthyroid and then becoming hypothyroid about six weeks after her thyroid was "killed."

Before she had RAI, Joan was eating constantly—and still losing weight. She was also extremely exhausted and learned that her heart rate was at a staggering high of 120 beats per minute. But after RAI, the weight started creeping back. Fatigue set in, and she felt achy. Sure enough, a TSH test showed that her levels were high. Her doctor put her on Synthroid, and her symptoms disappeared. She considers herself very lucky.

Although the prospect of becoming hypothyroid for life may seem unappealing, the alternative—not treating your overactive thyroid—is highly bothersome and potentially life-threatening. Keep in mind, too, that hypothyroidism is considerably easier to treat than hyperthyroidism is. The only challenge might be finding the right dosage, a process that may take some time and trial and error.

Antithyroid Drugs

Just as the name suggests, antithyroid drugs work in opposition to the thyroid. These drugs work by blocking the production of thyroid hormone by making it more difficult for the thyroid to use iodine. These drugs, which are called thionamides, have been around since the 1940s. Many patients are prescribed the drugs as the sole therapy for hyperthyroidism.

It can sometimes take several months for the effects of these medications to kick in. That's because the drugs do not wipe out the excess hormone already produced before you started taking the medication.

Most people who take medications for hyperthyroidism rely on PTU, which is usually taken three times a day. In addition to blocking the production of thyroid hormone, PTU blocks the conversion of T4 to the more active form of T3. The other option is methimazole, which is sold under the brand name Tapazole. Methimazole is usually taken daily or twice a day. For people living in Europe, carbimazole is another type of antithyroid medication that's available. In the body, carbimazole is rapidly converted into methimazole, where it blocks the production of thyroid hormone.

L. Essential

Antithyroid medications are usually given in the four to six weeks leading up to surgery for hyperthyroidism. They are also given in preparation for RAI in patients with severe hyperthyroidism. In addition, these drugs are used when someone has thyroid storm, a condition characterized by severe symptoms of hyperthyroidism and considered a bona fide medical emergency.

People who use antithyroid drugs usually stay on them for about two years. During that time, the dosage is adjusted so that your thyroid function gradually becomes normal. Approximately 20 percent of patients will have to discontinue the medication due to side effects such as a skin rash or nausea.

But for others, the antithyroid drugs can offer complete relief. After two years, approximately 50 percent of patients will be effectively cured, can stop the antithyroid drugs, and have normal thyroid tests. For the remaining 30 percent of patients who remained on the drugs, normal thyroid function is not achieved. Sometimes, the hyperthyroidism returns when the drugs are stopped. For these people, RAI or surgery becomes necessary.

Antithyroid Drugs Before RAI

Sometimes, doctors prescribe antithyroid medications to prepare patients for RAI. The drugs help bring the levels of thyroid hormone back to normal and reduce the odds of a sudden surge in hormone levels after RAI treatment. However, antithyroid drugs interfere with the uptake of iodine, so they're generally stopped two weeks before RAI.

Antithyroid drugs also interfere with RAIU and scans. That's why Dr. Friedman recommends performing RAIU and scans to determine the type of hyperthyroidism before starting antithyroid drugs. In the meantime, beta-blockers can be started immediately and can be used to tame symptoms of hyperthyroidism regardless of the cause.

Antithyroid Drugs Plus Thyroid Hormone

Some physicians may use a combination of an antithyroid treatment with thyroid hormone replacement. The antithyroid drug is given first to suppress the TSH and shut down the thyroid gland completely. It is then followed up with thyroid hormone replacement to gradually restore normal thyroid function. Some experts believe that the combination of the two drugs is more likely to induce a patient with Graves' disease into remission—a return to normal thyroid levels—than is antithyroid medication alone.

But not everyone is a good candidate for this combination therapy. Patients who are sensitive to either medication may be even more vulnerable to side effects when the drugs are given together. In addition, the combination is not suitable for patients who are sensitive to antithyroid drugs, since higher dosages are needed to completely suppress the thyroid gland.

Side Effects

As with any medication, antithyroid drugs can cause side effects. Some people may develop a low-grade fever at first that eventually subsides. Other side effects include a skin rash, itching, hives, hair loss, stomach upset, altered taste, tingling, joint pain and swelling, and nausea and vomiting. People who experience side effects may consider switching to the other drug but may experience similar problems with the second drug as well.

In rare cases, the antithyroid medications can produce major side effects. The most serious of these side effects is a decrease in the production of white blood cells, a condition known as agranulocytosis. This condition affects less than 1 percent of patients on antithyroid drugs and may be more likely to occur in older adults who take PTU or in people who take extremely high doses of methimazole.

 Alert

Antithyroid medications aren't the only drugs that can cause agranulocytosis. Anticonvulsants, used to control seizures, and certain antipsychotics, such as clozapine, can also cause a significant reduction in white blood cell production.

Agranulocytosis tends to occur in the first three months after starting treatment and is more common in patients aged forty and up. Because it is a possible side effect, it is important to tell your doctor about any sign or symptom that signals an infection such as unexplained fever or sore throat, or unusual bleeding or bruising. Your doctor will probably order a white blood cell count. Although the condition usually disappears once you discontinue the antithyroid drug, it is potentially deadly.

Other serious side effects of using antithyroid medications are liver damage from hepatitis, aplastic anemia, and vasculitis. In aplastic anemia, the bone marrow stops producing blood cells. With vasculitis, there is inflammation of the blood vessels. Fortunately, these side effects are exceedingly rare and tend to disappear fully once the drug is discontinued. But you should alert your doctor to any unusual signs or symptoms, including abdominal pain, yellowing of the skin or eyes, and loss of appetite.

Take Drugs Safely

Before using an antithyroid drug, it's important to tell your doctor about pre-existing medical conditions and other medications you are taking. The potency of these other medications as well as that of the antithyroid drugs can be altered when the medications are taken together. It's especially important to discuss anticoagulants, or blood thinners, such as warfarin (Coumadin); diabetes medications; and digoxin (Lanoxin), which is used to treat heart failure and abnormal heart rhythms. You should also tell your doctor about any vitamins and supplements you may be taking.

Essential

While the use of drugs is generally discouraged during pregnancy, some health conditions—including thyroid disease—require treatment for the healthy development of the fetus. Always discuss any drugs and supplements you use with your doctor, including over-the-counter products.

It's also important to tell your doctor if you are pregnant, plan to become pregnant, or are breast-feeding. Methimazole cannot be taken during pregnancy because it can prevent the normal development of the baby's thyroid. Also, babies breast-fed by moms on methimazole are at risk for hypothyroidism. But because hyperthyroidism is harmful to a developing fetus, you will need to take low doses of PTU. You will also require frequent monitoring. We'll go into more detail on your thyroid and pregnancy in Chapter 14.

What's Best for Each Condition?

Because there are such diverse options, it's important to have an understanding of the different treatments for the different types of hyperthyroidism. In general:

- If Graves' disease is the cause of your condition, medication or RAI is usually the top choice for treatment, then surgery.
- If you have toxic multinodular goiter, the best choice is RAI, followed by surgery, then medication.
- If hot nodules are the cause of your hyperthyroidism, RAI is generally the best treatment, followed by surgery.
- If you have thyroiditis, the best treatment is the passage of time, though you may need beta-blockers to tame your symptoms, and aspirin to reduce the inflammation.

Proper Dosing

Every patient starts on a dose that best fits her situation. The more severe your hyperthyroidism, the higher your dose will be. Once your thyroid function stabilizes, you may be placed on a maintenance dose to ensure healthy amounts of thyroid hormone. In general, if you are on PTU, you will need to take your pills more frequently than someone on methimazole would.

About four weeks after you start taking your antithyroid drug, your doctor should monitor your hormone levels. If they're still high, you may need to increase your dosage. However, if hormone levels have fallen significantly, you may be able to reduce the dose of your drug and prevent the onset of hypothyroidism. After these initial tests, you should be monitored regularly until your TSH levels are normal. Beyond that, you may still need to have your thyroid hormone levels checked to make sure the hyperthyroidism doesn't recur. Patients usually take antithyroid medications for up to two years, at which time they can taper off the dosage.

Be Consistent

Ideally, you should take your antithyroid drug at the same time every day and be consistent about how you take it. If you take it with food, then you should always take it with food. Don't take it with food one day and then on an empty stomach the next. Food affects the absorption of your medication, and being consistent day after day helps ensure that you have even amounts of the drug in your blood at all times.

If you happen to miss a dose, take it as soon as possible. If it's almost time for your next dose, then skip it and just take your next pill. You should not take a double dose to make up for one you missed.

Store It Properly

Many people stash their medications in the bathroom cabinet, where they're easily accessible in the morning or evening. But in reality, the bathroom isn't always the best place for drugs that need to be at room temperature.

Antithyroid drugs are best stored at room temperature in tightly sealed containers away from any moisture. Heat and steam from multiple showers can raise the temperature in a bathroom cabinet enough to affect the potency of the drugs stored there. Other storage places you need to beware of include kitchen cupboards near the stove or dishwasher, the glove compartment of your car, and a counter or window ledge that sits in direct sunlight. Instead, store antithyroid drugs at room temperature in a place that is removed from heat, light, and moisture.

Surgery

For most people with hyperthyroidism, surgery is usually a last resort. People usually turn to surgery if they don't want to take antithyroid drugs or undergo RAI treatment or have had limited success with the other two options.

Surgery may involve removing part of the thyroid gland, called a partial thyroidectomy. If only one lobe is removed, it is called a lobectomy. Surgery might also mean removal of the entire gland, which is called a total thyroidectomy. Partial thyroidectomy retains part of the thyroid, so you may not need thyroid hormone replacement for life. A total thyroidectomy ensures that you will not develop hyperthyroidism, but it does mean you will become hypothyroid.

L. Essential

Your ability to return to routine activities after surgery will depend largely on your level of discomfort. The one prohibition is swimming, which you cannot do until the incision is fully healed. You will be able to resume driving as soon as you can comfortably turn your head. Most patients can return to work within two weeks, and go back to leisure activities within a week.

Surgery is sometimes considered for women who are pregnant or planning to become pregnant. It may also be done in people with Graves' disease who have a large goiter that is obstructing breathing and swallowing. It may also be an option for people who have tried antithyroid medications without success and who cannot have RAI.

Side Effects

After surgery, you may notice some pain in your neck and some pain when swallowing. You may also experience some tension and stiffness in your neck. In addition, your voice may be hoarse. Most of these side effects are temporary and will disappear after about a week of normal activity.

Risks of Surgery

Like any surgical procedure, thyroid surgery comes with its share of risks. There is potential damage to the vocal cords and to the parathyroid glands, which are both located near the thyroid gland. Damage to the vocal cords can affect your voice, while damage to the parathyroid gland can lower blood levels of calcium, causing numbness, muscle pain, and depression.

The best way to prevent these risks is to choose an experienced surgeon, one who has done several surgeries on the thyroid. Do not hesitate to travel to locate a skilled surgeon. The expertise and abilities of a skilled surgeon will more than make up for the time and expenses involved.

Other Drugs

Figuring out how you're going to cure hyperthyroidism can take time. While you're at it, your doctor may prescribe other medications to treat your bothersome symptoms. After all, it can be exhausting to have an elevated heart rate and persistent tremors, and to live in a constant state of anxiety. The following section will discuss the different types of drugs your doctor may initially prescribe to relieve you of your symptoms.

Beta-blockers

These medications—known as beta-adrenergic receptor antagonists—are generally used to treat high blood pressure, relieve angina pain, and to prevent heart attack in people who have had previous attacks.

In people with hyperthyroidism, beta-blockers have a similar effect. Hyperthyroidism causes an increase in beta-adrenergic receptors in your body cells, which causes your cells to use more adrenaline, a hormone that speeds up your heart rate. Beta-blockers work by blocking the effects of adrenaline. They can slow a rapid heart beat, lower blood pressure, reduce tremors, and improve irregular rhythms of the heart. As a result, your heart requires less blood and oxygen and doesn't have to work as hard.

There are actually several different types of beta-blockers. Two of the most common ones used in hyperthyroidism are atenolol (Tenormin), which is given once or twice a day, and propanolol (Inderal), which is taken three to four times a day. Propanolol, but not atenolol, also blocks the conversion of T4 to T3, so you have less thyroid hormone available to body cells.

Certain people with pre-existing conditions should be careful about taking beta-blockers. Always tell your doctor if you have heart disease, heart failure, diabetes, depression, kidney disease, liver disease, or circulation problems. Beta-blockers can also aggravate several respiratory conditions such as asthma, emphysema, and severe allergies. If you have these pre-existing conditions, there's a chance your doctor may not use these medications.

Question

What can I do for insomnia caused by hyperthyroidism?
One option is to ask your doctor for a prescription sleep medication, such as Ambien (zolpidem). Like most sleep remedies, Ambien is recommended only for short-term use. Practicing good sleep habits, like going to bed on a regular schedule, exercising regularly (especially in the morning), and avoiding caffeine, can also help.

You should also be cautious if you are already taking other medications, since combining them with beta-blockers can affect the potency of one or both drugs. Drugs that warrant mention include hormonal contraceptives, diuretics, diabetes medications, heart medications, nonsteroidal anti-inflammatories, and calcium channel blockers.

While taking beta-blockers, you may experience side effects. Common ones include dizziness, fatigue, lightheadedness, upset stomach, and diarrhea. Some people may develop depression. More serious side effects are rare, but include swelling, shortness of breath, unusual weight gain, and fainting.

Iodine Solutions

As you already know, iodine has numerous uses in the diagnosis and treatment of thyroid disease. For people who have severe hyperthyroidism, these iodine solutions are sometimes used to temporarily block the production of thyroid hormone. These treatments include potassium iodide, sodium iodide, and Lugol's solution, which is sometimes simply called strong iodine. They are given in the short-term for a rapid reduction of symptoms.

 Fact

Lugol's solution was named after the French physician Jean Guillaume Auguste Lugol (1786–1851). The solution contains iodine, potassium iodide, and distilled water. He originally touted his solution as a treatment for tuberculosis (TB). Although it did not succeed in treating TB, Stanley Plummer did use Lugol's solution to treat hyperthyroidism.

The use of the iodine solutions is at the discretion of your doctor. Situations that may warrant their use include:

- Before surgery in Graves' disease to reduce blood flow to the diseased thyroid tissue.
- For treatment of severe hyperthyroidism or thyroid storm.
- After RAI in patients with Graves' disease who are allergic to antithyroid drugs, in order to normalize thyroid function.
- To relieve persistent mild hyperthyroidism in patients who have undergone RAI months earlier, in order to avoid a second dose of RAI.

Iodine solutions, however, should not be used in patients with a multinodular goiter. The additional iodine may only fuel the production of thyroid hormone.

Achieving Remission

The eventual goal of any treatment for hyperthyroidism is remission, in which the disease becomes inactive and the symptoms disappear. Physicians differ on how best to achieve this goal, and different patients will experience differing levels of success with the various treatments. Individual patients will also have personal preferences for how they are treated. Some may leap at the chance to put a permanent end to their hyperthyroidism with RAI, while others may prefer trying antithyroid medications first, in the hopes that the treatment will push them into a remission. Others choose medications in the hopes they will not become hypothyroid.

Many people with Graves' disease who try antithyroid medications do indeed go into remission. Those who are more likely to go into remission are usually people with mild hyperthyroidism, who have a small goiter, low levels of antibodies, and no eye disease. In rare cases of Graves' disease, your condition may go into remission on its own without treatment, a phenomenon known as spontaneous remission.

But in some cases, the remission is temporary, and the hyperthyroidism returns. If that happens, you will need to revisit your treatment options again and work with your doctor to devise a plan.

CHAPTER 9

Graves' Disease

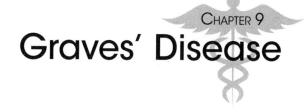

When the autoimmune system goes awry and attacks the thyroid, most people develop Hashimoto's disease as a result. A smaller percentage of these people develop Graves' disease, which is the most common cause of hyperthyroidism in the United States. In this chapter, you'll take a closer look at what Graves' disease is, including its causes, symptoms, diagnosis, and treatment options. You'll also learn what other autoimmune diseases to be on the lookout for as a person with Graves'.

What Is Graves' Disease?

Like Hashimoto's disease, Graves' disease is an autoimmune disease, a condition caused by an immune system that mistakenly attacks its own healthy tissue. In healthy people, the immune system is on duty 24/7, always on the lookout for invaders like bacteria and viruses that threaten your health. When an invasion occurs, your immune system generates antibodies that attack the invaders, called antigens. The white blood cells work feverishly to destroy the invaders and bring about healing.

When someone has an autoimmune disease, these white blood cells are mysteriously summoned for no apparent reason, and the body treats normal healthy tissue as something foreign. The body then begins to produce antibodies against the perceived invader. Antibodies produced in an autoimmune disease are known as autoantibodies.

In people with Graves' disease, the most common antibodies are the TSI antibodies and the TPOAb. TPOAb are the same antibodies that cause Hashimoto's disease, which was discussed in Chapter 6. Graves' disease was named after Robert Graves, an Irish doctor who first identified the condition in three of his patients in early 1835.

Fact

A British physician named Caleb H. Parry first noted the constellation of symptoms now known as Graves' disease in the 1780s. In the 1840s, a German physician named Baron Carl Adolph von Basedow also devoted much study to the same condition. Although the disease is primarily called Graves' disease, some people may know it as Basedow's syndrome or Parry's disease.

An autoimmune attack can occur in various organs and body systems, each causing its own disease and constellation of symptoms. In Graves' disease, your thyroid is the organ under siege. As a result of this autoimmune attack, your thyroid is enlarged and churning out way too much thyroid hormone, producing the symptoms you know as hyperthyroidism. The enlargement of the thyroid gland has earned the disease the name of diffuse toxic goiter.

Unlike Hashimoto's disease, Graves' is less common and occurs in about 1 percent of the U.S. population. The condition is eight times more common in women than men and is more likely to occur in adults in their thirties and forties. The disease is much less common in adults over age fifty.

Causes and Symptoms

No one knows exactly what causes the body's immune system to turn against its own healthy cells in Graves' disease or any other autoimmune condition. One thing we do know is that the condition definitely has a tendency to run in families.

Because autoimmune problems are much more prevalent in women, some experts think hormones may be involved in the disease process, too. But as with most other autoimmune conditions, no one knows for sure how reproductive hormones might promote autoimmunity.

Some experts suspect that environmental factors are at play as well. One study in 2005 found that cigarette smoking was linked to the incidence of Graves' in women—the more cigarettes women smoked, the greater their likelihood of developing Graves'.

Other studies have suggested that emotionally stressful events may play a role in triggering Graves' disease. Still other possible culprits include viruses, infections, pollution, and bacteria. But again, these are theories, and the exact cause of any autoimmune disease remains a mystery. Most people believe that it's a combination of genetics and environmental factors that cause Graves'.

Essential

It is possible to have no symptoms of hyperthyroidism and still have Graves' disease. Most people who have this condition, which is called euthyroid Graves' disease, have thyroid eye disease. Some become hyperthyroid, but others never do.

In mild cases, Graves' disease sometimes produces no symptoms at all, especially in the early stages. But in most people, though not all, Graves' disease tends to lead to symptoms of hyperthyroidism. Eventually, you may begin to notice that you're losing weight for no apparent reason despite an increase in appetite. Your heart may be beating faster, and you may feel nervous and on edge.

You may also be sweating more often and sensitive to warm temperatures that others find comfortable. Women may notice that their periods are lighter or that they disappear altogether.

As your body's metabolic rate increases, you may have more frequent bowel movements, possibly even diarrhea. You may also notice hair loss and rapid growth of your fingernails. Your skin may be more delicate and thin, and you may notice trembling in your hands. At night, you may be plagued by insomnia. By the end of the day, you are frequently exhausted.

Too much thyroid hormone also takes a toll on your moods. Besides feeling anxious and jittery, you may be irritable, quarrelsome, and sad. Your moods may swing wildly for no apparent reason, and you may fluctuate between bouts of depression and mania. In some people, Graves' disease can resemble panic disorder.

Unfortunately, the antibodies involved in Graves' disease attack the eyes, too. As a result, Graves' disease affects the eyes in a way that other forms of hyperthyroidism does not, although people who have advanced hyperthyroidism of any type will appear to have a wide-eyed, startled appearance. This unusual stare occurs when the muscles that raise the upper eyelid are overstimulated by the excess thyroid hormone, causing the skin of the upper eyelid to be slightly lifted, exposing the white above the top of the iris. About half of people with Graves' will go on to develop a separate condition called thyroid eye disease, or infiltrative ophthalmology. The condition is also sometimes called exophthalmos. With this condition, patients develop a distinct bulging of the eyeball. This protrusion occurs as a result of swelling in the muscles around the eyes, which pushes the eyeball forward. Some people may have difficulty closing their eyes completely, which leads to redness and irritation of the eyeball. You will find a more thorough discussion of thyroid eye disease later in this chapter.

Diagnosis and Treatment

Determining whether you have Graves' disease involves a physical exam and a discussion of your symptoms. While the symptoms you reveal to your doctor may immediately suggest hyperthyroidism, changes in your eyes and an enlargement of your thyroid are usually the telltale signs that indicate you have Graves' disease and not a form of thyroiditis, which is an inflammation of the thyroid.

To confirm that you have Graves' disease, however, your doctor will want to order blood tests. Low levels of TSH, combined with high levels of free T4 and free T3, will indicate that you do, indeed, have hyperthyroidism.

Tracing the cause of hyperthyroidism to Graves' disease, however, requires other tests. Often, diagnosis also involves an RAIU test that can help confirm Graves' disease. This test involves ingesting a small amount of RAI. Hours later, a camera is placed in front of your neck to see where the iodine is concentrated. In people with Graves' disease, the RAIU test will reveal that the thyroid is absorbing a lot of iodine to produce thyroid hormone. The scan will show diffuse uptake of iodine over the whole gland.

Sometimes, doctors will check the blood for specific autoantibodies. The most telling substances in the blood are the TSIs. These are sometimes referred to as thyroid-stimulating antibodies (TSAs) or thyroid receptor antibodies (TRAb). These antibodies behave like TSH and will bind to TSH receptors in the thyroid gland, prompting them to produce thyroid hormone. But unlike TSH, TSIs do not stop the production of thyroid hormone once the levels get too high. TSIs are also responsible for thyroid eye disease.

People who have Graves' disease also have other autoantibodies in their blood, namely TPOAb and TgAb. Both these autoantibodies are also present in people with Hashimoto's disease, which makes them less conclusive than the TSI antibodies. TPOAb affects the thyroid by attacking the enzyme involved in iodine uptake. TgAb destroys thyroglobulin, the protein that stores thyroid hormone. Experts believe that these antibodies are present in low levels in about 10 percent of the population but do not cause any signs or symptoms.

Treating Graves' disease typically involves the options outlined in the previous chapter. The goal is simple: to restore thyroid hormone levels to normal. You may have RAI treatment to destroy the diseased thyroid tissue or take antithyroid drugs in the hopes of inducing a remission. Surgery is usually a last resort.

Essential

Some people with Graves' disease may describe manic behavior. But unlike true mania, which causes a real increase in your energy levels, hyperthyroidism in Graves' disease tends to bring on exhaustion.

Some people with Graves' disease will go into remission without medication. But this is extremely rare and occurs primarily in cases where the disease is mild.

Any course of treatment has advantages and disadvantages. Finding the perfect amount of RAI, for example, is often very difficult. High doses of RAI are more likely to be successful but almost guarantee that you'll be hypothyroid in the end. But giving patients a more conservative amount of RAI often doesn't work. Too little treatment, and you wind up still battling hyperthyroidism.

If you opt to take antithyroid medication, you may be able to avoid hypothyroidism, but you may continue having symptoms of hyperthyroidism. To help you decide, you should review your options carefully with your doctor and weigh the advantages and disadvantages of each treatment. Your decision will also be influenced by several other factors, including personal preference, allergies to medications, previous health conditions, and whether you are pregnant.

Thyroid Eye Disease

The eyes are often involved in people who have Graves' disease. The same antibodies that trigger hyperthyroidism attack the tissues of the eyes, causing inflammation, swelling, and bulging. These symptoms produce a condition called thyroid eye disease, or Graves' ophthalmolopathy or Graves' orbitopathy. It is also sometimes called exophthalmos.

Although the majority of people with Graves' disease have some eye involvement, the severity varies widely. In general, people who smoke tend to have greater eye involvement. Many people develop eye problems well in advance of hyperthyroidism, while others start having eye problems after they are diagnosed with Graves'. In some cases, you may have eye problems without hyperthyroidism.

In the absence of hyperthyroidism, however, many people mistake the symptoms of thyroid eye disease for infection or other eye problems. Symptoms of thyroid eye disease include:

- Redness and irritation
- Gritty sensation, itchiness, or watery eyes
- Sensitivity to light or sun
- Dry eyes
- Lid lag, in which the upper eyelid is slow to close when your gaze is down
- Wide-eyed stare
- Bulging of the eyes
- Double vision or diminished vision

All these symptoms are believed to be the result of an attack by the same antibodies that affect the thyroid. These antibodies appear to stick to eye muscles, causing them to swell and become inflamed. Once the eyes are inflamed, they may remain that way for months, even years.

Thyroid eye disease is most common in middle-aged adults. If it does occur in older adults, it can be more severe. The condition is rare in children and teens. Some people believe that stress plays a significant role in predicting who gets thyroid eye disease and the severity of it.

When it's mild, treating thyroid eye disease often focuses on symptom relief. Artificial tears sold in drugstores can help lubricate dry and irritated eyes as can cool compresses applied to the eyes. Relief also means taking steps to shield your eyes from irritating situations. Try to avoid bright sunlight and areas that are drafty, windy, or smoky, which can aggravate your eye condition. When you do go outside, wear wraparound sunglasses to shield your eyes from the light.

Alert

The use of RAI to treat hyperthyroidism may worsen thyroid eye disease in some patients. The worsening of the symptoms is most pronounced in people who smoke and in people with severe hyperthyroidism. It is also more likely in people who have previous eye problems and patients with high levels of autoantibodies. Some studies have suggested that steroids such as prednisone given before and after RAI can prevent worsening of eye symptoms.

At night, you may want to try sleeping on extra pillows or elevating the head of your bed, so you can reduce the swelling in your eyes. Place a humidifier in the bedroom to help minimize dryness. And drink plenty of water throughout the day to help your eyes stay hydrated.

If the disease becomes more severe, you may need a steroid such as prednisone to help reduce the pain, swelling, and inflammation. The use of steroids, however, must be closely weighed against the drug's side effects, which include weight gain and a higher risk for infection. Also, steroids do not correct bulging of the eyes.

In extreme cases, in which the swelling becomes severe, you may require surgery to correct the eyes. A procedure called orbital decompression surgery can sometimes help patients whose eyeballs are bulging so badly that they are at risk for vision loss. Before surgery, your surgeon will order an MRI to see the extent of your eye disease. The surgery involves removing bone from the eye socket in order to make room for the excess tissue. Another option is external beam radiation, which uses X-ray beams to reduce inflammation in the back of the eyes.

If thyroid eye disease causes serious cosmetic problems, you may want to consider plastic surgery to alter the appearance of the eyes. In some cases, eyelid surgery may be done to correct eyelids that no longer close properly, and eye muscle surgery may be considered to correct misalignment of the eyes. Double vision can also be corrected with the use of eyeglasses that contain a prism. Regardless of what you do to correct your eye problems, if you have Graves' eye disease, your endocrinologist and ophthalmologist will have to work closely together to decide your best course of treatment.

Skin Problems

In rare instances, Graves' disease can affect the skin and cause Graves' dermopathy. The condition develops as a result of a buildup of protein in the skin.

The two most common types of skin problems are pretibial myxedema (PTM) and thyroid acropachy. People who develop PTM will develop a thickening of the skin, usually on the front of the lower leg or on the tops of the feet. The affected area resembles an orange peel, and may appear as raised patches of pink skin. PTM occurs in less than 5 percent of Graves' patients—mostly women. It is primarily a cosmetic problem and is usually treated with steroid creams.

Thyroid acropachy is even rarer than PTM and occurs in just 1 percent of people with Graves' disease. With thyroid acropachy, the hands and fingers develop a clublike appearance. Occasionally, the toes are involved, too. The condition is more common in people who develop PTM and in people who smoke.

Treatment of hyperthyroidism in Graves' disease usually helps reduce both skin conditions.

Other Issues

Like Hashimoto's disease, having Graves' disease can raise your risk of developing other autoimmune diseases. Autoimmune diseases tend to run in families. Having one condition puts you at risk for others.

Although the majority of people with Graves' disease will not develop any other disorders, it's important to know what some of these autoimmune conditions are in case you do start to experience symptoms. Keep in mind, too, that you may be more likely to develop Graves' disease if you have one of these other conditions. (See Chapter 6 for a more thorough discussion of these conditions.)

Having Graves' disease can also make it hard for women to get pregnant. You may not even be ovulating. In addition, it puts you at risk for having a baby with birth defects. It also increases the likelihood for miscarriage and premature labor and delivery.

If you have Graves' disease and you want to get pregnant, it's best to wait until the condition is under control before attempting to conceive. Trying to treat Graves' during pregnancy can be difficult, and some treatments, such as RAI, are potentially harmful to the fetus.

If, however, you develop Graves' disease while you are pregnant, you will need to consult with both an endocrinologist and your obstetrician-gynecologist to devise a safe treatment plan. Many women with hyperthyroidism wind up taking low doses of propylthiouracil (PTU), without causing harm to their baby. Doses that are too high can cause goiter and hypothyroidism in your baby.

The natural tendency of the immune system in pregnancy is to become less active, so that the developing fetus is not rejected. For a woman with Graves' disease, this slowdown of the immune system can provide a welcome, albeit temporary, reprieve. We'll take a closer look at pregnancy and your thyroid in Chapter 14.

Goiters and Nodules

CHAPTER 10

A goiter is an enlarged thyroid gland, and a nodule is a lump. Think of goiters and nodules as signs that something may be going on in your thyroid gland. But like any kind of thyroid disease, it takes some medical investigation to find out what's going on. In this chapter, we'll take a look at these two irregularities of the thyroid gland, including how to spot them and the treatment options available for each.

What Is a Goiter?

A goiter is an enlarged thyroid gland. Thanks to the introduction of iodized salt in the 1920s, goiters have become much less common in North America than they once were. But goiters can still occur as the result of conditions other than iodine deficiency.

The word *goiter* comes from the Latin word *guttur*, which means "throat." Having a goiter doesn't mean that the amount of thyroid hormone in your body is too high, too low, or normal. It just means that the gland is bigger than it should be, and that there may be a disease process going on that's causing the problem. In reality, there are many different ways to describe goiters, depending on whether nodules are present, how many there are, and whether you have any other symptoms:

- Diffuse goiters are smooth and uniformly large.
- Nodular or multinodular goiters are lumpy and characterized by the presence of one or more nodules.

- Toxic goiters, sometimes called thyrotoxic goiters, are those that occur with hyperthyroidism.
- Nontoxic goiters are those that do not involve abnormalities in thyroid hormone production or malignancy.
- Toxic multinodular goiters comprise numerous nodules and cause hyperthyroidism.
- Sporadic nontoxic goiters occur in people with healthy thyroid function. The goiter may be diffuse, nodular, or multinodular.

Worldwide, the primary cause of goiter is iodine deficiency. Iodine, as you know by now, is a critical ingredient in the production of thyroid hormone. According to the Thyroid Foundation of America, nearly a quarter of the world's population do not get enough iodine in their diets. For these people, large goiters are common and often occur with nodules and severe hypothyroidism.

Without enough iodine, your thyroid works extra hard to make the thyroid hormone that your body needs. This added effort causes the thyroid gland to get bigger.

Fact

The International Council for the Control of Iodine Deficiency Disorders (ICCIDD) was created in 1985 for the sole purpose of achieving optimal iodine nutrition worldwide. The goal of eliminating iodine deficiency is done primarily through universal salt iodization. Currently, about 70 percent of households worldwide consume iodized salt. And countries such as China, Thailand, and Peru that were previously iodine deficient are significantly improved. Regions of the world that are still lagging include Central Asia and Africa.

Although the introduction of iodized salt in the United States has significantly lowered the incidence of goiter caused by iodine deficiency in this country, goiters still occur. In some cases, albeit much less commonly, goiters can be caused by excess iodine in the diet.

Goiters are also caused by hypo- and hyperthyroidism. In people with underactive thyroids, inadequate amounts of thyroid hormone cause TSH levels to go up, spurring the development of a goiter. In the United States, goiters associated with hypothyroidism are most often caused by Hashimoto's disease. Goiters may also be the result of an overactive thyroid brought on by Graves' disease, which causes the gland to swell and enlarge.

In people who develop toxic multinodular goiters, the progression of disease usually follows a common course. It typically starts when someone from an iodine-deficient area develops a goiter. Over time, nodules begin to form in the goiter. Eventually, one or more nodules becomes autonomous, and toxic multinodular goiter develops.

These events may take decades to unfold, which is why toxic multinodular goiter is more common in older patients. You are also more likely to get toxic multinodular goiters if you move from an iodine-deficient region, like the mountainous areas of Mexico, to an iodine-sufficient place like the United States. The shock of eating iodine-rich foods after years of not having enough iodine causes nodules to become autonomous and produce their own thyroid hormone.

In some cases, a goiter can simply occur on its own, in the absence of any malfunction of the thyroid gland. These are sometimes called euthyroid goiters. Some people develop a goiter when they have thyroiditis, inflammation of the thyroid gland.

Evaluating Goiters

Deciding how to treat a goiter involves first figuring out what caused the enlargement. Your doctor will want to know the symptoms you've been experiencing and your family history for thyroid and autoimmune diseases and also whether you have a personal or family history of thyroid cancer. Your doctor may also ask if you've ever been exposed to external radiation.

Alert

People who have had previous thyroid problems such as nodular goiters, Hashimoto's or Graves' disease should be careful about ingesting too much iodine. Excess iodine in the diet can raise your risk for hypothyroidism and hyperthyroidism.

In addition, your doctor will do a physical exam of your thyroid area. One test he might perform is a Pemberton's maneuver. During this exam, you will be asked to stand and face him. While looking ahead, you will be asked to raise both arms straight into the air, with both arms near the ears. If your neck turns red, the veins in your neck bulge, and you start to have difficulty breathing, the test will suggest an obstructive goiter, one that is big enough to block the area between the neck and chest and interfere with breathing, swallowing, and blood flow.

TSH Test

A blood test to measure your TSH level will help your doctor determine whether you have hyperthyroidism or hypothyroidism. Elevated levels of TSH suggest that you are hypothyroid, meaning the pituitary gland is producing more TSH in an effort to get the thyroid to make more thyroid hormone. Low levels indicate you have hyperthyroidism and excessive amounts of thyroid hormone. TSH tests can be followed up with autoantibody tests to determine whether you have Hashimoto's or Graves' disease.

Ultrasound

An ultrasound of the goiter can reveal its size, whether it contains nodules, and whether those nodules are solid or cysts. Over time, ultrasound can reveal whether the nodules are getting bigger and whether a goiter has formed.

RAIU and Scan

When a goiter is associated with symptoms of hyperthyroidism, an RAIU and scan may be done to see where iodine is being taken up. This test is often done in patients with toxic multinodular goiters. Places where the scan is brighter reveal the presence of hot nodules, which absorb more iodine. These hot nodules are never cancerous. Nodules that are dark are considered cold but may sometimes harbor cancerous cells.

Treatment for Goiters

The type of treatment you receive for a goiter will depend on the size of the goiter and the symptoms associated with it. Small goiters that are causing no problems often require no treatment at all. Goiters that are bigger and causing symptoms, however, do require medical attention. Large, unsightly goiters may even require cosmetic surgery to improve the patient's appearance.

Ⓔ Essential

In rare cases, a goiter may grow downward into the chest cavity, causing a substernal goiter that rests against the lungs, trachea, and blood vessels. A substernal goiter may cause coughing and a sensation that something is stuck in the throat. Some people may notice solid foods getting trapped in the upper esophagus and difficulty breathing and lying on their back. Treatment usually involves surgery to remove the thyroid gland and goiter.

Often, treatment of the underlying problem—such as hyperthyroidism or hypothyroidism—is enough to shrink the goiter. (See Chapters 5 and 8 for specific treatments.) With patients who have euthyroid goiter, some doctors may try giving what is called levothyroxine suppressive therapy, which suppresses TSH levels. But levothyroxine suppressive therapy rarely works, and most patients wind up with hyperthyroidism.

Toxic Multinodular Goiters

Treating a toxic multinodular goiter is somewhat trickier. Unlike the goiters that occur in Graves' disease, toxic multinodular goiters do not go into remission and don't respond to antithyroid medications. Instead, treatment typically involves RAI or surgery to definitively remove the goiter.

Sometimes, patients with a toxic multinodular goiter will not have the ability to take up high levels of RAI, the way diseased thyroid tissue in Graves' disease does. This situation can make it hard for the goiter to absorb the RAI that is necessary to kill the diseased tissue. In these cases, patients may be pretreated with lithium or recombinant TSH to enhance iodine uptake and RAI treatment. RAI may be especially useful in elderly patients and others in whom surgery is considered high risk.

Most patients treated with RAI for toxic multinodular goiter often get only an ablation of their hot areas. Since the remaining tissue is not affected by the disease process, hypothyroidism is not likely to occur.

But in some patients, surgery may be the only alternative. People who have large goiters that are causing compression, for example, are good candidates for surgery. Surgery is also used in cases when RAI is impractical or has been ineffective.

Nontoxic Goiters

Often, nontoxic goiters cause no symptoms at all, so no treatment is required. Some doctors may use RAI or surgery, especially in cases where a nontoxic goiter causes compression or is large. In patients with nontoxic goiters who receive RAI, the goiter can sometimes shrink. In general, the higher the uptake of iodine, the more likely the goiter will shrink.

Thyroid Nodules

Simply put, a nodule is a lump. The vast majority of thyroid nodules are small, benign, and harmless. They may occur as a single nodule or as a clump. By some estimates, nodules occur in as much as half the population, often without symptoms or problems. Nodules are more common in women than men, and become more common with age.

Essential

Nodules are very common, especially among older adults. Among all adults aged fifty, half will have at least one thyroid nodule, according to EndocrineWeb.com. Among adults aged sixty, 60 percent will have at least one thyroid nodule. And in adults aged seventy, 70 percent will have at least one thyroid nodule.

Many people won't even notice they have a nodule until their doctor feels one in their throat during a routine physical. But if the nodule gets bigger, you may actually be able to see it on your throat as a lump in the lower front of your neck. Women may notice it when they're applying makeup or face cream. Men may feel it while they're shaving or notice that their shirt collars are becoming uncomfortably snug. Large nodules may actually press against your windpipe or your esophagus, making it difficult for you to breathe or swallow. Sometimes, these larger nodules can affect your voice and cause hoarseness.

Types of Nodules

At first glance, all nodules appear the same. But in reality, there are several different types of nodules. Some cause no problems, while others may cause minor problems. Still others can get rather large and churn out their own thyroid hormone, causing hyperthyroidism. The three main types of nodules are:

- **Toxic Adenomas:** Also known as autonomous toxic nodules, toxic adenomas develop as a result of a genetic mutation in the thyroid follicular cell. Toxic adenomas produce their own thyroid hormone and can cause hyperthyroidism. We'll discuss these in more detail later.
- **Cysts:** Cysts account for 15 to 25 percent of all nodules. Most cysts are filled only with fluid. Those that contain solid material as well as fluid are known as complex cysts. Large ones may need ongoing monitoring and evaluation.
- **Colloid Nodules:** Colloid is the substance at the center of a thyroid cell. A colloid nodule is made up mostly of colloid. It is always benign and usually does not produce much, if any, thyroid hormone.

Nodules can produce annoying symptoms, but the vast majority of nodules are benign, with only a small percentage turning out to be malignant. For example, a single nodule in an otherwise healthy gland is more likely to be cancerous than a multinodular goiter. A nodule that is hard to the touch is another sign that your nodule may be cancerous. Nodules accompanied by enlargement of the lymph nodes in the neck may also indicate cancer. The bottom line is this: All nodules warrant medical attention and evaluation to pin down the exact cause and type of nodule.

A Look at Toxic Adenomas

Of all the different types of nodules, the ones that cause the most severe hyperthyroidism are the toxic adenomas, which develop as a result of an abnormality in the follicular cell of the thyroid. Normally, TSH receptors in the follicular cell require TSH to turn on the cell and trigger the production of thyroid hormone.

With toxic adenomas, a mutation causes the TSH receptor to be permanently turned on, even without TSH. As a result, thyroid hormone is produced in excess, and the cell multiplies and divides, eventually causing a nodule to form.

Evaluating Nodules

Some nodules cause pain. Others may cause swelling. Still others cause no symptoms but can be felt by an experienced physician. In any case, if a nodule is detected in your thyroid gland, it's critical to get a thorough evaluation of the nature of the nodule and whether it's cancerous or not.

 Alert

Statistically speaking, malignant nodules are more likely to occur in children, adolescents, and men than they are in women. You're also at greater risk if you received radiation treatments in the 1940s and 1950s for conditions such as acne or tonsillitis. In addition, a single lump is more likely to be malignant than are several nodules.

Several tests can help your doctor determine whether the nodule is benign or malignant, active or inactive. These include:

- **Fine Needle Aspiration (FNA):** Aside from surgery, an FNA is the only way to determine whether a nodule is cancerous or not. Doing an FNA involves retrieving cells from the nodule, which are then studied closely for cancer. Sometimes, a diagnosis cannot be made after an FNA, and the procedure must be repeated.
- **Ultrasound:** An ultrasound of the nodule can reveal its size and whether it is solid or a cyst. Over time, ultrasound can reveal whether the nodules are getting bigger.
- **RAIU and Scan:** An RAIU and scan may be done to see whether your nodule is hot. A hot nodule appears brighter on the scan, showing that the nodule is taking up iodine for the autonomous production of thyroid hormone.
- **TSH Test:** Measuring the level of TSH in your blood can reveal whether a hot nodule is causing hyperthyroidism. When the

level of TSH is suppressed, it confirms that you have a toxic adenoma.

Sometimes, in spite of all these tests, a physician cannot say for sure whether a nodule is benign or malignant. Some may be benign, but others may be precancerous, meaning they'll eventually become cancer if they're left untreated. Still others may actually be cancer. The problem is that no test can definitively prove that the nodule is benign, and nothing can demonstrate that the nodule is positively cancerous. In these cases, the nodules are deemed suspicious, and treatment usually involves surgery.

Treatment for Nodules

Deciding on a course of treatment depends on whether the nodule is benign or malignant, as well as whether it's toxic or not. The size of the nodule also matters. In this section we'll deal with benign nodules. Chapter 11 is devoted exclusively to thyroid cancer and will explore your treatment options for thyroid cancer in greater detail.

As you've read, a small colloid nodule that is causing no problems generally doesn't require any treatment. But if a nodule gets too big, it can cause serious problems. At night, you may have trouble breathing when you lie down and the nodule presses against your windpipe. At meals, you may have trouble swallowing foods because the nodule is up against your esophagus. In some cases, a large nodule may become unsightly, making you self-conscious about your appearance. All of these situations may mean that surgery is needed to remove the nodule.

Treating Indeterminate Nodules

When a nodule is indeterminate, you will probably undergo surgery. Removing the half of the thyroid gland that contains the nodule is considered the safest course of action, in the event the nodule is cancerous. Doing surgery also brings you closer to an answer to the nagging question: is it cancer? Close examination of the removed tissue can then help determine whether there is indeed cancer. If the doctor does find malignancy, you may need to undergo further surgery to remove the entire thyroid gland.

Treating Cysts

Although cysts are sometimes quite small, they can grow rapidly and unexpectedly and cause pain and discomfort. For this reason, most cysts are treated with aspiration, a technique in which the fluid inside the cyst is drained with a syringe. The problem with aspiration is that the cyst often recurs, and may even come back bigger than before. In that case, a second aspiration is required. Some doctors may use ethanol in the treatment of cysts after the fluid is drained. Under the guidance of a special needle, ethanol is injected into the cyst, causing the walls of the cyst to stick together and erode the inner space of the cyst. Studies have found that using ethanol with aspiration is more effective than aspiration alone.

Treating Toxic Adenomas

Your TSH is suppressed, and you definitely have a hot nodule churning out excess thyroid hormone. For some people, a toxic adenoma causes symptoms of hyperthyroidism, such as nervousness, trouble breathing, and a rapid heart rate. If you're experiencing symptoms of hyperthyroidism, your doctor may prescribe a beta-blocker to control your symptoms until you treat the nodules.

To actually treat the toxic adenomas, however, you will need RAI or surgery since these nodules will not go into remission, even with the help of antithyroid drugs. The dosage of RAI used with toxic adenomas is slightly higher than that used in treating Graves' disease, but it is lower than the amount used to treat thyroid cancer. You'll know that you got the right dosage if thyroid hormone levels start to dip in a few weeks, and then TSH starts to rise, as the pituitary gland begins responding to the lower amounts of thyroid hormone in the body.

For some people, RAI is not a good option. People with extremely large toxic adenomas, who are pregnant, or who have had no success with RAI may need to consider surgery instead. Surgery usually involves removing all or part of the thyroid gland. Even if you remove only part of the thyroid gland, you will probably need to take thyroid hormone replacement after surgery. The medication will stabilize the production of thyroid hormone and help ensure that the nodule does not recur.

CHAPTER 11

Thyroid Cancer

These days, everyone lives in fear of the C word—cancer—a disease that has wreaked havoc on millions of lives. In people who have thyroid cancer, the prognosis is good: most people are successfully treated and live long, productive lives. Nonetheless, thyroid cancer is a serious condition, and in the aftermath of treatment, requires lifelong vigilance and care. In this chapter, you'll learn what thyroid cancer is, how to detect it, and how it's treated.

What Is Thyroid Cancer?

Cancer is a common condition these days. According to the American Cancer Society, nearly half of all men and a third of all women will have some form of cancer in their lifetime. As of 2001, there were approximately 9.8 million Americans still living who had a history of cancer. Cancer is the second leading cause of death in the United States, just behind heart disease.

Any form of cancer is serious, but if you're destined to get cancer, thyroid cancer is one of the better ones to get. Most people are successfully treated and do not die of thyroid cancer.

Like other kinds of cancer, thyroid cancer is the growth of abnormal cells. Unlike healthy, normal cells, these abnormal cells do not die out but multiply, spawning more and more abnormal cells that eventually overwhelm healthy functioning of an organ and spread elsewhere. Fortunately, in most cases of thyroid cancer, these abnormal cells grow relatively slowly.

The Mysterious Cause

The cause of cancer is still largely a mystery. But scientists do know that the root cause is damage to the DNA (deoxyribonucleic acid), the genetic material in every single body cell that carries the instructions for nearly everything our cells do. In a lifetime, it's normal for DNA molecules to experience some damage. Most times, the cell can repair itself. But in cancer cells, the damaged DNA goes unrepaired, and the abnormal cells grow, often causing a malignant, or cancerous, tumor.

A patient's symptoms, treatments, and prognosis depend a great deal on where the cancer is located. Your chances for survival also depend in large part on how early the cancer is detected and treated.

 Alert

A nodule or lump in the thyroid is one sign that you may have thyroid cancer. But keep in mind that as many as 95 percent of these nodules are benign. See your doctor if you feel or see anything suspicious in your neck.

In people who have thyroid cancer, the prognosis is generally good. According to estimated predictions from the American Cancer Society, approximately 25,690 cases of thyroid cancer were expected in 2005. Of those, 19,190 were expected to occur in women, and 1,490 were expected to eventually be fatal. In other words, only one of sixteen cases of thyroid cancer lead to death due to the cancer. The key is early detection, particularly of unusual lumps and nodules in the thyroid gland.

Who Gets Thyroid Cancer?

Too much sun raises your risk for skin cancer. Smoking cigarettes makes it more likely you'll develop lung cancer. But when it comes to thyroid cancer, there are few specific risk factors that make one person more likely to develop thyroid cancer than the next person. Most people who have thyroid cancer have no apparent risk factors, and some who have at least one risk factor never get the disease.

One factor that does raise your risk of thyroid cancer is exposure to radiation. People who were exposed to radiation in childhood seem more likely to develop thyroid cancer as adults. Years ago, radiation was used to treat acne, fungal infections of the scalp, enlarged tonsils, and adenoids in children. (Note: This type of radiation is different from routine X-rays.) As adults, these people have a higher risk of thyroid cancer. Exposure to local radiation as adults, however, does not appear to be linked to thyroid cancer.

Exposure to radiation from nuclear fallout such as at Chernobyl also increases your risk. The Ukrainian city of Chernobyl was the site of a major nuclear power plant accident in 1986. Many children living in that area went on to develop thyroid cancer. Adults involved in the subsequent cleanup also have a higher than normal rate of thyroid cancer.

Here in the United States, some studies have found a higher incidence of thyroid cancer—as well as other thyroid diseases—in people living near certain nuclear facilities, such as the Hanford nuclear processing facility in Richland, Washington, and testing sites for nuclear bombs in regions such as that outside Las Vegas, Nevada.

Fact

According to the American Cancer Society, the incidence of thyroid cancer has been increasing in both sexes since 1980, although the increase is larger in women than it is in men. Between 1980 and 1998, the incidence for men and women combined increased at an average of 2.5 percent per year. Since 1998, thyroid cancer incidence has been increasing at an average of 7.7 percent annually.

Another risk factor is family history. Approximately 5 percent of people who develop papillary thyroid cancer have a relative who had the disease, too. And approximately 20 percent of cases of medullary thyroid cancer are the result of an abnormal gene that is inherited from a parent.

Thyroid cancer is also more prevalent in women than it is in men. Elsewhere in the world, thyroid cancer is more common among people who eat a diet low in iodine. But some people, like Pat, had no risk factors and no signs or symptoms.

Pat learned she had thyroid cancer during a routine doctor visit when her physician felt a lump. She had noticed nothing at all. She decided to have her entire thyroid removed, which turned out to be a good decision. During the surgery, the surgeon found a second tumor on the other side of her thyroid.

Detecting Thyroid Cancer

Most people have no symptoms of thyroid cancer. Those who do have symptoms, however, may notice a lump in their neck that appears to be getting larger. You may also notice pain in the front of your neck or that your voice is suddenly hoarse for no apparent reason. Some people experience difficulty swallowing or have trouble breathing easily. In others, thyroid cancer may cause a constant cough that doesn't go away. All of these symptoms warrant medical attention and immediate biopsy.

Finding a lump in your throat might be frightening. Keep in mind, however, that most lumps or nodules are benign and noncancerous. The only way to know for sure is to see your doctor as soon as you can. Your doctor will do a physical exam and ask you about your medical history and family history. Your doctor will also need to perform some tests. The most important one is the FNA biopsy.

Fine Needle Aspiration (FNA) Biopsy

The simplest and most direct way for detecting thyroid cancer is with an FNA of the lump or nodule. The FNA is the key to diagnosing thyroid cancer. It is an office procedure that involves using a thin needle to obtain cells from the nodule, which are then examined by a pathologist for cancer.

To perform this test, your doctor will have you lie down, with your neck extended backward and a pillow under your shoulder for comfort and support. Local anesthesia is sometimes applied to the area over the nodule, though some patients may not want any anesthesia at all. A thin needle is then inserted into the nodule for several seconds and cells are withdrawn.

This procedure can tell you whether the lump is cancerous or benign. If the nodule is cancer, the FNA can reveal what kind of cancer it is.

Alert

If you don't like needles, ask your doctor for a sedative before a biopsy. Some patients may be given a drug such as Valium to ease their worried minds. You might also want to practice deep breathing or meditation to help you stay calm.

The procedure is often repeated several times so that cells can be collected from different parts of the nodule. The cells are then sent to a lab and examined by a pathologist. Most times, the FNA is highly accurate in diagnosing papillary and medullary thyroid cancers. But in people who have follicular thyroid cancer, an FNA is often not accurate or is inconclusive. If the biopsy shows follicular cells, the patient may go for surgery, or the nodule may be watched for several months to see if it grows. A nodule that is rapidly growing is likely to need surgery.

Sometimes there may not be enough cells in the aspirate—the substance collected by this needle—and the biopsy is called nondiagnostic. In that case, the FNA needs to be repeated.

Ultrasound

Physicians often use ultrasound to help diagnose thyroid cancer. An ultrasound is helpful in determining the size of the nodule and how many nodules there are. In addition, ultrasounds are helpful in determining whether a nodule is fluid filled or solid. Both types can be thyroid cancer.

Many doctors use ultrasound at the time of the FNA to assist in the placement of the needle. An ultrasound is also used after a portion of the thyroid has been removed, when scarring from the surgery has made it more difficult for your doctor to examine your remaining thyroid gland.

An ultrasound is done using a transducer wand. Jelly is applied to the region being examined, in this case the neck. The transducer is then moved along the neck, creating sound waves that form an image of your thyroid on a computer screen. The procedure is painless and not invasive.

Ultrasounds can be effective at finding cancer after the thyroid gland is removed if the cancer comes back in the neck or elsewhere in the body. But an ultrasound image is by no means conclusive. It only provides evidence that there may be a recurrence of cancer and that a biopsy is needed. Sometimes, tiny nodules are found by ultrasound but do not need to be biopsied.

Thyroid Scan

Nuclear imaging is undoubtedly an invaluable tool in diagnosing and treating thyroid diseases. But in people with thyroid cancer, a thyroid scan is mostly used to determine whether the cancer has spread.

Most types of thyroid scans involve two steps: the scan itself and an RAIU test. For the procedure, you will be given a pill or an injection that contains RAI. Several hours later, a camera is placed in front of your neck to take a picture of where the iodine is concentrated in your neck. You may also get a test called a thyroid uptake that measures the amount of radiation taken up by the thyroid.

 Fact

There are two types of iodine used for thyroid scans. Iodine-123 and 131. Generally, I-123 has a shorter half-life and leaves the body sooner. But I-131 may be more effective because it stays in the tumor longer. Scans may also be done with an element called technetium.

Areas of the thyroid that do not take up iodine are considered cold nodules because they do not show radioactivity. Nodules that have absorbed iodine will turn up as hot nodules. Hot nodules may occur in hyperthyroidism. The problem with the thyroid scan as a diagnostic tool in cancer is that virtually all nodules, both malignant and benign, appear cold, making it impossible to distinguish the benign from the malignant.

But thyroid scans are of use in patients who have had their thyroid glands removed because of papillary or follicular thyroid cancer. Any remaining cancer cells will take up the radioactive iodine and appear on the scan. Thyroid scans are not used for medullary forms of thyroid cancer since the cancer cells in that disease will not absorb iodine.

Other Diagnostic Tools

FNA and ultrasound are the primary ways for diagnosing thyroid cancer. But your doctor may use other tools as well to help determine whether the cancer has spread. For example, your doctor may use computerized axial tomography (CAT) scans. CAT, or CT, scans are advanced X-rays that shoot several beams from different vantage points, which are then viewed on a computer screen, not film. The

CT scan gives you a glimpse of the surrounding muscles, including the trachea, the esophagus, and the lymph glands.

Your doctor may also use magnetic resonance imaging (MRI), which uses a magnet to create vibrations in a targeted area, then produces a detailed image on a computer. Like the CT scan, an MRI can tell you the size of a thyroid nodule and whether it has spread to other parts of the body.

If you have a difficult or aggressive tumor, your physician may recommend a positron emissions tomography (PET) scan. PET scans of the thyroid require the use of radioactive glucose.

Essential

Besides cancer, PET scans are used to help diagnose neurological problems, including Alzheimer's disease. In people with Alzheimer's, a PET scan will show less activity in certain parts of the brain than that which occurs in a healthy person.

Because thyroid cancer cells have a faster metabolism than normal cells, they will take up the glucose at a more rapid rate. The radioactivity is then seen with the use of special scanning equipment and used to form an image of the tumors in the body. PET scans are just starting to be used by doctors, but may be useful for detecting recurrent cancer and to pinpoint the spread of cancer.

Types of Thyroid Cancer

Thyroid cancer doesn't occur in just one form. In fact, there are actually four distinct types of thyroid cancer, depending on where the cancerous cells develop. These different types of thyroid cancer span the whole range of cancer experience, from the tiny, slow-growing papillary form to the aggressive and fast-growing anaplastic form, a rare but deadly variation of thyroid cancer. Figuring out the type of cancer you have is the first step toward getting proper treatment.

Papillary Thyroid Cancer

The vast majority of thyroid cancers are papillary carcinomas. This type of thyroid cancer originates in the thyroid follicle cells and usually grows very slowly. In fact, papillary cancer grows so slowly that microscopic cells of this kind of cancer are found in 6 to 35 percent of autopsies, even though the person died of another cause.

In most cases, the cancerous cells occur in just one lobe of the thyroid, though they may occur in both lobes in 10 percent of the cases. Most people develop papillary thyroid cancer before age forty, and the majority of cases have no symptoms.

In some cases, a physician can detect papillary thyroid cancer just by feeling a lump in the thyroid gland. Some people may notice an enlarged lymph node or gland in their neck.

Fact

Little Orphan Annie was a comic strip created by Harold Gray in 1924. Annie was based on a character from a nineteenth-century poem by James Whitcomb Riley. It was the unusual appearance of her eyes—drawn as empty circles—that attracted the attention of medical experts, who noted the resemblance to thyroid cancer cells.

In any case, papillary thyroid cancer occurs within the nucleus of the thyroid cell. A healthy nucleus appears dark and round under a microscope. Cancerous nuclei show up as large, clear, circular areas that resemble what some describe as Little Orphan Annie eyes, after the 1920s comic-strip character. These cellular changes are called optically clear nuclei and are a key to diagnosing papillary thyroid cancer. Some nuclei may appear to have a line or groove through them, which is also an indication of papillary thyroid cancer.

Follicular Thyroid Cancer

The second most common kind of thyroid cancer is follicular thyroid cancer. This type of cancer accounts for about 20 percent of all cases of thyroid cancer. It is a more aggressive form of thyroid cancer and tends to occur in slightly older people. Although follicular thyroid cancer is less likely than papillary cancer to spread to the lymph nodes, it is more likely to enter the bloodstream and metastasize to other organs, such as the lungs, bladder, and liver.

Follicular thyroid cancer usually appears as a painless lump in the thyroid. But diagnosing follicular thyroid cancer is difficult. An FNA is generally unable to determine whether the lump is cancerous. Some characteristics of the nodule may appear suspicious, in which case, the doctor will do surgery to remove the nodule and have it examined by a pathologist for cancer.

Some people may develop a subtype of follicular thyroid cancer called Hurthle cell carcinoma, or oxyphil cell carcinoma. This type of cancer accounts for 4 percent of all thyroid cancers. In people with Hurthle cell carcinoma, the thyroid loses its ability to take up iodine, making it hard to use radioactive iodine in treating this form of cancer.

Another type of follicular thyroid cancer is insular thyroid cancer. This form of cancer is more aggressive than ordinary follicular thyroid cancer, but may still take up RAI.

Medullary Thyroid Cancer

Remember the parafollicular cells—also called C cells—tucked between the thyroid cells? As you might recall, these cells produce a hormone called calcitonin, which is involved in regulating calcium in your body. When cancer cells grow in the parafollicular cells, it is called medullary thyroid cancer.

These cancers account for 5 percent of all thyroid cancers. About 20 percent of people with this form of thyroid cancer inherited it from a parent. Anyone who has medullary cancer should have their parathyroid glands and adrenal medulla screened for tumors because medullary cancers may be associated with tumors in these glands, as described below.

⌐ Essential

> Medullary thyroid cancer that has spread cannot be effectively treated with chemotherapy. It also can't be treated with RAI therapy since the cancerous cells don't take up iodine. The only option is a total removal of the thyroid and usually the lymph nodes as well.

Medullary cancer is relatively easy to diagnose. That's because the cells make calcitonin. Calcitonin then enters the bloodstream and can be detected by a simple blood test. There are essentially four types of medullary thyroid cancer (MTC):

Sporadic MTC

Most cases of medullary thyroid cancer are called sporadic MTC. This form occurs in people who have no family history of the disease. It occurs most often in older adults and typically involves just one lobe.

Inherited MTC

This less common form occurs in each generation of a family. If it's the only type of cancer in the family, it's called isolated familial medullary thyroid carcinoma (FMTC). The familial forms of MTC often develop in childhood or early adulthood. Besides the isolated form, you could have one of two other subtypes, which involve tumors on other endocrine organs:

MEN2A

MEN stands for "multiple endocrine neoplasia," which refers to tumors elsewhere in the endocrine system. If you have FMTC as well as tumors of the adrenal and parathyroid glands, you are said to have MEN2A. Tumors of the adrenal medulla, called pheochromocytomas, produce adrenaline, while tumors of the parathyroid gland cause elevated blood-calcium levels.

MEN2B

People with MEN2B have tumors of the adrenal gland but no problems with the parathyroid gland. Rather, they experience benign growths called neuromas on their tongue, the underside of the eyelids, and throughout the gut. People with MEN2B often have thick lips and thick eyelids as well as elongated fingers and toes.

Anaplastic Thyroid Cancer

Anaplastic thyroid cancer is relatively rare and accounts for about 2 percent of all thyroid cancers. Experts believe it develops out of an existing papillary or follicular cancer that, for unknown reasons, spins out of control. But it is an extremely aggressive form of cancer that rapidly invades the rest of the neck, then spreads to other parts of the body. The condition is also sometimes called undifferentiated thyroid cancer.

 Fact

Former Chief Justice William Rehnquist died of anaplastic thyroid cancer in September 2005, just eleven months after he was diagnosed. Early on, he was given a tracheotomy—a hole in the windpipe—to alleviate an obstructed airway and to make breathing easier. The procedure is highly unusual in thyroid cancer and signaled the seriousness of his condition.

This form of thyroid cancer is more common in older people, and like the other kinds, occurs more often in women than men. But unlike other forms, the symptoms are abrupt and obvious. Patients often have trouble breathing and changes in their voice, such as hoarseness, caused by the fast-growing cancer pressing against their windpipe. Most patients will also see a large lump in the front of their neck.

Unfortunately, most people with anaplastic thyroid cancer will die within a few months of diagnosis, unless it is caught in its very early stages. Less than 10 percent of people who have it will survive more than five years.

Thyroid Lymphomas

Lymphomas are cancers that grow out of lymphocytes, the primary cell type in the body's immune system. Lymphomas usually start to grow in the lymph nodes. Thyroid lymphomas are rare and account for only about 3 percent of thyroid cancers. They usually occur in older adults who have Hashimoto's disease. Thyroid lymphomas usually begin as a fast-growing nodule.

Treatment for Thyroid Cancer

When it comes to thyroid cancer, the primary treatment is surgery. But the amount of surgery that is performed depends on the type of cancer you have.

In cases where the cancerous nodule is small and confined to one lobe, you may have just one lobe removed, which is known as a lobectomy. If the tumor is large and has spread to both lobes or beyond the thyroid gland, the surgeon will remove the entire thyroid, a procedure known as a total thyroidectomy. Some surgeons will perform a subtotal thyroidectomy, in which the surgeon removes most of the thyroid but leaves some tissue around the parathyroid glands and the important nerves. This is done to avoid damaging the parathyroid gland and nerves. Each patient's circumstances will vary, and you will need to discuss your treatment options closely with your doctor.

Thyroid surgery for cancer usually takes about two hours and requires a hospital stay of three to seven days. Although rare, you may experience some complications such as temporary or permanent hoarseness, excessive bleeding or infection of the wound, and numbness or tingling. In extremely rare cases, you may suffer damage to the parathyroid glands, which can lower blood-calcium levels and result in muscle spasms.

Essential

When choosing a thyroid surgeon, look for experience. According to the New York Thyroid Center, a skilled surgeon will do at least fifty thyroid or parathyroid surgeries a year. The surgeon's practice should concentrate on these types of operations.

After surgery, you will be placed on thyroid replacement hormones to replace what your body no longer makes. The dose of replacement hormones is often high enough to help keep your TSH levels low, too. Too much TSH has been known to provoke cancer cells, though it does not affect people with medullary cancer.

Staging Your Cancer

After it's been determined that you have cancer, the next step is figuring out what stage it's at. Staging helps your doctor determine future treatments. The stage you're at depends on your age, the size of the tumor, and whether it has spread.

In your research, you may come across different staging systems. But all of them follow about the same pattern. People who are younger and have smaller tumors are generally at the earlier stages of cancer and have higher chances of survival. People who are older and who have larger tumors are considered to be in the more advanced stages and have a reduced chance for survival.

In patients where the cancer has spread, the prognosis is worse than it would be if it had stayed local. The good news is, most patients can still be treated and survive.

℧ Question

What is the five-year relative survival rate?
This phrase refers to the percentage of patients who are still alive at least five years after their cancer is diagnosed. When they say early-stage papillary thyroid cancer patients have a five-year relative survival rate of 100 percent, it means 100 percent of those diagnosed in a given year are still alive five years later.

RAI Therapy

In most people, surgery is supplemented with RAI therapy. RAI is used to destroy any lingering thyroid tissue that was not removed by surgery or to treat thyroid cancer that has spread to other parts of the body. RAI is the only way to kill cancer cells in the thyroid gland without causing harm to other parts of the body.

Before receiving RAI, you will be asked to temporarily discontinue your thyroid hormone pills and eat a diet low in iodine. That's because you need high levels of TSH in order for the therapy to be most effective. Without enough thyroid hormone, your pituitary gland will produce more TSH, which, in turn, will encourage the papillary and follicular forms of cancer to take up the RAI that destroys them. The low-iodine diet is needed so that ingested iodine does not interfere with the iodine in the RAI.

The first dose of RAI is called the ablation dose, and it is usually given about six weeks after surgery to wipe out any remnants of thyroid tissue. After that, your doctor will determine your schedule of RAI treatments and how long you will need them. Some treatments for cancer will require a two- or three-day hospital stay, but others can be done on an outpatient basis.

In cases where the cancer has spread to other organs, patients may be given lithium before and after RAI. Lithium is best known as a treatment for bipolar disorder. In thyroid cancer, lithium enhances the effects of the RAI in cancer cells outside the thyroid, causing the RAI to remain in the cells for a longer duration.

After receiving high doses of RAI, you may be required to stay in an isolated room so that your radioactivity does not harm other people, including the hospital staff. Items in the hospital room may be covered in protective material so that patients who stay in the room after you do not become contaminated.

Upon discharge, you will be told to take precautions for several days so that you do not contaminate others. Here's a list from the AACE:

- Use private toilets, and flush twice after each use.
- Bathe daily and wash hands frequently.
- Use disposable eating utensils or wash yours separately.
- Sleep alone, and avoid prolonged close contact.
- Launder your linens, towels, and clothes daily and separately from others.
- Do not prepare food for others that requires prolonged handling.
- Steer clear of small children.

The rigors of these guidelines can temporarily change your life. Janet, for example, sent her family to live with her parents.

During this time, Janet covered the furniture she used with sheets, ate off of paper plates, and wore latex gloves the entire time. She also confined herself to two rooms. Before her family returned, she did numerous loads of laundry and wiped down all the surfaces. She recalled the experience as rather strange.

Some people will experience permanent side effects from RAI. You may notice tenderness in your neck, nausea, stomach irritation, and dry mouth. Some women may notice that their periods become irregular, and men who receive large doses may be at risk for infertility. Women of childbearing age are advised not to get pregnant for six months to a year after RAI treatment.

Essential

If you've been asked to cut back on iodine for an upcoming RAI treatment, check out the Low-Iodine Cookbook online at the Thyroid Survivors' Association, Inc.'s Web site, at *www.thyca.org*. The free cookbook features 185 recipes from the Thyroid Cancer Survivors' Association, Inc. volunteers as well as strategies for eating less iodine. Remember, all foods that list salt as an ingredient also contain iodine.

Other Treatments

If your cancer has spread to other organs or if you have medullary cancer that does not take up iodine, you may be given external beam radiation therapy or chemotherapy. External radiation involves a focused beam delivered from a machine outside the body. The powerful X-rays target and destroy the cancerous cells. Treatment is usually given five days a week for about six weeks. In some cases, the radiation can damage healthy tissue nearby. Some people also experience severe fatigue and temporary damage to the skin.

Chemotherapy involves anticancer drugs that are injected into the body or taken orally. The drugs enter the bloodstream, where they circulate throughout the body. The problem is, chemotherapy can often damage healthy cells along with the cancerous cells. The damage may put you at risk for infection, bleeding, and fatigue. You may also experience side effects such as nausea and vomiting, loss of appetite, hair loss, and mouth sores.

Monitoring and Follow-up

People who have had thyroid cancer must undergo regular monitoring to make sure the cancer does not return. Routine blood tests are also done to make sure you're on the proper amount of thyroid hormone replacement. As we said, that usually means a low TSH level. In people with medullary cancer, blood tests can reveal higher-than-normal levels of calcitonin.

Any abnormalities in the blood should prompt your doctor to do imaging tests to look for cancer. If the cancer does recur, you may need more surgery, RAI, radiation, or chemotherapy, depending on the location of the cancer and the extent of its spread.

To figure out whether your cancer has come back, your doctor may perform a thyroglobulin test and/or a whole body scan. Both tests require that you have elevated levels of TSH to stimulate any lingering thyroid cells—cancerous or not—to produce thyroglobulin or take up the RAI.

Thyroglobulin Tests

Normal healthy thyroid glands produce a protein called thyroglobulin (Tg). Anyone who has had a total thyroidectomy should have very little Tg in her blood. If it does show up in normal or high amounts, it can mean a return of cancerous thyroid cells, which will require further testing.

A single abnormal test, however, is not a definite sign of cancer. Whether the Tg levels rise steadily over time is more important, so your doctor may do more than one test. Also, some thyroid cancer patients may produce antibodies to thyroglobulin (TgAb), which can interfere with the test results. For that reason, your doctor may test for TgAb too. Most people who have had thyroid cancer will be tested for Tg annually.

Whole Body Scans

After your thyroid has been removed, your doctor may perform a whole body scan to look for recurrent thyroid cancer. To prepare for this procedure, you will need sufficiently elevated TSH levels and low levels of ordinary iodine in your body.

Alert

> When you do discontinue your thyroid hormone therapy, make sure to take measures to ensure your safety. Do not operate a car or any heavy machinery, and if possible, take time off from work. Do not use this time to do anything that requires a lot of mental effort or energy.

Until recently, raising your TSH levels—either for testing or for RAI treatment—required that you stop taking your hormone treatments and go into a state of hypothyroidism, sometimes for several weeks. For many people, this was rather uncomfortable. Now, there are two ways to raise your TSH levels that are less bothersome. Since 1998, most doctors have been using a drug called Thyrogen to raise TSH levels without discontinuing hormone therapy. Thyrogen is a synthetic version of TSH that has the same effect on lingering thyroid cells—it encourages them to take up the RAI, which makes them visible on the scan. However, Thyrogen is used only for diagnostic testing such as whole body scans and not for RAI treatment for cancer.

Another way to lessen the symptoms of hypothyroidism involves taking Cytomel (T3) six weeks prior to receiving the RAI. Two to three weeks before the RAI, you will discontinue the Cytomel.

After you are suitably prepared, and your TSH levels reach the required levels, you will undergo the whole body scan. For the scan itself, you will take a pill or injection that contains a small dose of RAI. You will then be scanned for cells that have taken up the RAI. The doctor will also test your Tg level at that time.

Whole body scans are used for detecting the recurrence of thyroid cancer or metastasis and use a much lower dose of RAI. You do not need to take measures to isolate yourself or shield others from radioactivity after the scan as you do when you get a high-dose RAI treatment.

Taking Care of Yourself

A great deal of follow-up cancer care rests with you, the patient. Follow your doctor's instructions closely on taking your medications and staying on a schedule of regular blood tests and checkups. Be vigilant about any changes in your body, and report them promptly to your doctor. If you're having a difficult time coping with the rigors of cancer treatment or surviving cancer, consider seeking out a mental health professional for counseling. Your state of mind will influence how well you fare after diagnosis and treatment for thyroid cancer, too.

We want to emphasize that it's very rare to die of thyroid cancer. Most people go on to live normal lives. The key is staying on top of your care.

CHAPTER 12

Thyroid Disease and the Endocrine System

The thyroid gland doesn't work in isolation but is part of an elaborate network of glands known as the endocrine system. Because these glands depend on each other for proper functioning, what happens in one can affect the others. This chapter will tell you how some glands can affect the thyroid and how thyroid disease can affect a major aspect of a woman's endocrinology—her monthly menstrual periods.

The Endocrine System

Think of the endocrine system as the body's communications network, where glands house hormones that act as chemical messengers and transmit information to cells throughout the body. These hormones influence almost every single body cell and organ and are responsible for growth, metabolism, and sexual development and function. Once released by specific glands, hormones travel through the bloodstream to the targeted organ, where they incite the organ to action. In addition to the thyroid, the endocrine system includes the:

- **Adrenal glands:** These are located above the kidney, and affect metabolism, the body's stress response, and salt regulation.
- **Hypothalamus:** This part of the brain regulates the pituitary gland as well as involuntary body functions, sleep, appetite, and hormones.

- **Ovaries and testicles:** These are the sex organs, which produce hormones involved in influencing female and male sexual characteristics. They regulate the menstrual cycle in women and sperm production in men.
- **Pancreas:** This is located below your stomach, and secretes insulin, a hormone that regulates the body's use of glucose.
- **Parathyroid glands:** These are located near the thyroid, and regulate calcium levels in the blood.
- **Pineal gland:** This is in the back of the brain, and produces melatonin, a hormone involved in sleep-wake cycles.
- **Pituitary gland:** This is located near the base of the brain, and produces numerous hormones that affect the other endocrine glands, including the thyroid.
- **Thymus gland:** This is located at the top of the chest, and is involved in the body's immune function.

Each one of these glands plays a vital role in keeping you healthy, but none of them exists in isolation. A problem in any of these glands can produce effects elsewhere in the endocrine system, including in the thyroid gland. The pituitary gland and the adrenal glands, in particular, have a direct connection to the thyroid.

Hypopituitarism

The pituitary gland is at the helm of the endocrine system and impacts everything from a woman's monthly menstrual cycle to one's ability to handle stress. This pea-sized gland, which is nestled at the base of the brain, is responsible for the secretion of several hormones that, in turn, trigger the release of other hormones. When the pituitary gland is diseased, the entire endocrine system is potentially affected.

Fact

Pituitary tumors are extremely common. Studies have found that benign tumors in the pituitary gland are present in about 25 percent of the population. To figure out the scope and significance of these benign brain tumors, Congress passed the Benign Brain Tumor Cancer Registries Amendment Act in October 2002. The law forces hospitals, clinics, and doctors to report pituitary tumor incidence rates in their cancer registries.

Sometimes, the pituitary gland may become underactive, causing a condition called hypopituitarism. This condition affects the anterior (front) lobe of the pituitary gland, which results in partial or complete loss of functioning in that lobe. As a result, the pituitary loses its ability to produce certain hormones. Symptoms of hypopituitarism will vary depending on which hormones are affected. The symptoms may develop slowly and gradually, or occur suddenly from seemingly out of nowhere.

Central Hypothyroidism

When hypopituitarism affects the pituitary's production of TSH, you may develop central hypothyroidism. Symptoms of central hypothyroidism are similar to those in hypothyroidism—you may experience weight gain, fatigue, depression, forgetfulness, and sensitivity to the cold.

Like hypothyroidism, central hypothyroidism can be difficult to diagnose. Despite the presence of symptoms, TSH levels are often in the low normal range. A more accurate measure may be free T4 levels, which are often low in people with central hypothyroidism. Doctors also rely on symptoms reported by the patient, which lead to testing for a deficit in several pituitary hormones.

Other Problems

The thyroid gland isn't the only gland that can be affected by hypopituitarism. Pituitary dysfunction may also cause a reduction in the production of several other hormones:

Growth Hormone (GH)

GH controls bone and tissue growth and maintains the appropriate balance of muscle and fat tissue. In adults, the lack of GH can cause fatigue, poor physical and mental function, and muscle weakness. In children, insufficient GH can stunt growth.

Luteinizing Hormone (LH)

LH regulates the menstrual cycle in women and stimulates testosterone production in men. Without enough of it, women may stop menstruating, become infertile, and experience vaginal dryness. In men, LH stimulates the production of testosterone, a hormone responsible for masculinization and libido. Without adequate LH, they experience erectile dysfunction.

Follicle-Stimulating Hormone (FSH)

FSH controls sperm production in men and ovulation in women. A deficiency causes a decrease in sperm production that can cause infertility.

Adrenocorticotropic Hormone (ACTH)

ACTH stimulates the adrenal glands to produce cortisol, the major stress hormone. Without it, you may experience weight loss, fatigue, depression, nausea, and vomiting.

Antidiuretic Hormone (ADH)

ADH regulates urine production and maintains water balance in your body. Inadequate amounts of ADH can cause diabetes insipidus, a condition characterized by excessive urination and thirst.

Prolactin

Prolactin regulates the development of female breasts, as well as the production of breast milk in nursing moms. Insufficient prolactin can make it hard for new moms to nurse.

As hypopituitarism gradually worsens, the number of hormones affected can increase, too, causing more symptoms. The hormones that are affected seem to follow a predictable pattern. The first hormone involved is usually GH, followed by LH and FSH, then TSH, and finally ACTH.

Causes

Many factors can trigger hypopituitarism. Causes include tumors, radiation, brain surgery, inadequate blood supply to the pituitary, infection, or head trauma. In some cases, the cause of hypopituitarism is an indirect problem with the hypothalamus, such as a tumor, TB, or sarcoidosis, an autoimmune disease that causes inflammation in the lungs and/or lymph nodes.

Diagnosis and Treatment of Hypopituitarism

Diagnosing hypopituitarism involves medical detective work to determine the cause of your hormone deficit(s). When several glands are underactive, it may suggest hypopituitarism. To make the diagnosis, your doctor will do a complete exam that includes your medical history and may also perform a CT scan or MRI to look for physical abnormalities in the pituitary gland. He will also order blood tests to measure hormone levels. Some of these measurements may require stimulation testing, in which hormones are given to see how the pituitary responds and which hormones are released.

Ĺ. Essential

One type of surgery for pituitary tumors is called transphenoidal hypophysectomy. The procedure involves removing the tumor through a cut in the nasal passage. More recently, the surgery has been done endoscopically, with a small tube going to the pituitary, which is then viewed through a microscope. The surgery does not cause scarring and usually involves little pain, but it does not correct hypopituitarism.

Treatment for hypopituitarism depends largely on the cause of the disease. If a tumor is found, for instance, you may need surgery, radiation therapy, or drugs to remove the tumor or shrink it. Regardless of whether surgery is needed, the goal of treatment is to replenish the body with the missing hormone(s). In people who have central hypothyroidism, that might mean taking thyroid hormone replacement.

The Adrenal Gland Connection

You've been diagnosed with hypothyroidism and put on levothyroxine. But for some reason, instead of feeling better, you feel worse. You've developed joint and muscle pain and a string of colds that you can't seem to shake. You are nauseous and have started vomiting. You wonder if something else may be going on. For some people, treating hypothyroidism may worsen a problem called adrenal insufficiency, in which the adrenal glands are not producing enough of certain adrenal hormones. In fact, untreated hypothyroidism may hide the symptoms of adrenal insufficiency.

The adrenal glands are located right above the kidneys, where they produce several important hormones. The inner medulla of the adrenal glands produces epinephrine and norepinephrine (adrenaline). The outer cortex of the adrenals produces several hormones, including cortisol, aldosterone, testosterone, DHEA, and estrogens.

The adrenal hormones play an important role in handling stress by providing the body with the chemical support it needs when you need to react quickly, what is commonly known as the "fight or flight" response. In times of stress, the hypothalamus releases corticotrophin-releasing hormone (CRH), which stimulates the pituitary to secrete ACTH. In turn, ACTH triggers the adrenal glands to release cortisol. Cortisol and adrenaline help the body brace itself to fight or flee by temporarily improving strength and agility, bolstering concentration and reaction time, and mobilizing reserves of fat and carbohydrates for immediate energy. In addition, these hormones are involved in several other bodily functions, including weight control, heart function, blood pressure, the balance of fluids, and blood flow to the muscles.

Fact

In the mid-nineteenth century, when Dr. Thomas Addison first identified adrenal insufficiency, the primary cause was tuberculosis (TB), a highly contagious bacterial infection of the lungs. Autopsies showed that TB was present in 70 to 90 percent of all cases. These days, TB accounts for roughly 20 percent of all cases of adrenal insufficiency.

In people who have adrenal insufficiency, these hormones are lacking. Some patients may be deficient in several hormones, while others may be deficient in just cortisol or just aldosterone, the hormone that regulates salt. If you also have hypothyroidism, it's been suggested that adrenal insufficiency can make it hard to treat your thyroid disease. More importantly, treating hypothyroidism can exaggerate adrenal insufficiency. The result is a highly uncomfortable constellation of symptoms.

Details of Adrenal Insufficiency

People who have adrenal insufficiency have many of the same symptoms as those who have hypothyroidism. They're tired, depressed, and weak. They may have joint and muscle pain and may sleep poorly. They may also have dry skin. The difference is patients with adrenal insufficiency tend to lose weight and get dehydrated, while hypothyroid patients gain weight and retain fluids.

 Alert

> People with an aldosterone deficiency should avoid low-salt diets. In fact, some need to be on a high-salt diet. Low aldosterone causes the kidneys to excrete excess salt, which lowers blood volume. The reduction in blood volume is especially hard on the brain. Without enough blood reaching the brain, patients are often fatigued and may experience a drop in blood pressure when they stand up.

In addition, people with adrenal insufficiency may have trouble recuperating from colds and illnesses, and have low blood pressure and low blood sugar. They're frequently dizzy when they stand up, and may have nausea, vomiting, and diarrhea. After a while, they may lose weight and notice a darkening of their skin. They may also develop cravings for salty food. In people who have hypothyroidism as well, these symptoms worsen once they start taking thyroid hormone replacement.

Causes

It's rare for the adrenal glands to go haywire. When they do, it can sometimes be a problem with the glands themselves, which can reduce both the amount of cortisol and aldosterone. In some cases, an adrenal problem is actually a problem with the pituitary gland, which reduces the amount of ACTH the pituitary releases and hampers the production of cortisol. Several diseases and events can cause adrenal insufficiency, including:

- Addison's disease (primary adrenal insufficiency), which is most often caused by an autoimmune attack on the adrenals
- Congenital adrenal hyperplasia, an inherited disorder characterized by a deficiency in cortisol and, in some cases, aldosterone. The condition occurs because an enzyme that produces cortisol is not working properly, and therefore the synthesis of cortisol is blocked
- Surgical removal of the adrenal glands
- Surgical removal of the pituitary gland

In some cases, adrenal insufficiency is a temporary medical problem brought on by infection or surgery to remove a tumor from the pituitary gland or adrenal glands. Treatments to reduce elevated cortisol levels found in Cushing's syndrome can also trigger a temporary bout of adrenal insufficiency.

Diagnosis and Treatment

Making a diagnosis for adrenal insufficiency isn't always easy. The symptoms often develop gradually and sometimes are not serious enough for the patient to seek treatment. In about 25 percent of cases, it isn't until the patient develops acute adrenal insufficiency that treatment is sought. When adrenal crisis—sometimes called Addisonian crisis—occurs, symptoms are much more severe and may include abdominal pain, severe vomiting and diarrhea, dehydration, low blood pressure, and loss of consciousness. Without immediate treatment, an adrenal crisis can be fatal.

Fortunately, most people do get medical help before a crisis occurs and will report their symptoms to their doctors. To determine if you have a problem, your doctor needs to measure the amount of ACTH coming from the pituitary and the amount of cortisol being produced by the adrenals. Hormone levels are best measured in blood tests. Many patients also need a stimulation test called a cosyntropin test to make the diagnosis. Measuring blood renin and aldosterone is often helpful, too. Renin, a substance produced by the kidneys, helps regulate aldosterone.

Alert

Anyone who has adrenal insufficiency should wear a medical brace-let and carry a syringe prefilled with steroids. Adrenal crisis is usually brought on by infection, trauma, or severe stress. The best strategy is prevention and recognizing the subtle symptoms of deficiency.

Treatment for adrenal insufficiency depends on the cause of your condition, but almost everyone requires daily medication to keep the condition under control. In an adrenal crisis, patients may need to administer their treatment by injection.

To replace cortisol levels, you may need to take hydrocortisone, prednisone, or dexamethasone, which are synthetic glucocorti-coids, or steroids. If you're deficient in aldosterone, you may need a drug called fludrocortisone (Florinef). As with thyroid hormone replacement therapies, it can sometimes take time to find the right dose, so you may go through a trial period before you do. The dos-ages may also need to be adjusted during times of stress since your body won't naturally produce these hormones in response to crisis. In some cases, your doctor may also ask you to increase your salt consumption.

The Thyroid Link

For the thyroid, the depletion of adrenal hormones can have profound effects, most notably the worsening of symptoms. Some experts believe that the adrenal hormones play a role in the conver-sion of T4 into T3.

Having hypothyroidism can sometimes reveal an underlying problem with adrenal insufficiency. If you are taking thyroid hor-mone replacement but do not notice an improvement in your symp-toms—or you experience a worsening—ask your doctor to check your adrenal glands. You may need simultaneous treatment of both your thyroid and adrenal glands.

Establishing the proper balance of these two treatments is tricky. It often takes some time and effort on both your part and that of your doctor to find the ideal balance of the two treatments. But the effort is well worth it when both conditions are successfully treated.

Thyroid and Menstruation

In healthy women, the menstrual cycle is simply an accepted fact of life, a monthly event that sometimes brings on temporary mood swings, fatigue, and cravings for high-fat foods. But many women endure monthly challenges with their menstrual cycle. They may have periods that are heavy, irregular, or extremely painful. In some women, their periods are fine for years, and then suddenly become problematic.

Fact

In the United States, the average age a girl starts menstruating is twelve, but it can start as early as eight or as late as sixteen. On average, menstruation will stop and menopause will occur when a woman is around age fifty-one.

When something is irregular with the menstrual cycle, most women don't look to their thyroid as the culprit. Instead, they may blame stress, a recent illness, or advancing age. They may think they're having early signs of menopause. But often, the real reason for their menstrual problems is their thyroid.

The Inner Workings of Menstruation

Menstruation is a monthly event that prepares a woman for pregnancy. In the first half of the menstrual cycle, levels of estrogen rise, causing the lining of the uterus to grow and thicken. The rise in estrogen is followed by an increase in FSH, which triggers an egg, or ovum, in one of the ovaries to start to mature. At about day fourteen of a typical twenty-eight-day cycle, there is a surge in LH, and the egg leaves the ovary, an event known as ovulation.

During the second half of the menstrual cycle, the egg travels through the fallopian tube to the uterus in anticipation of fertilization. In preparation, progesterone levels rise to help prepare the uterine lining for pregnancy. If the egg becomes fertilized by a sperm cell and attaches itself to the uterine wall, the woman becomes pregnant.

But most times, the egg is not fertilized, and simply dissolves or is absorbed into the body. If pregnancy does not occur, estrogen and progesterone levels drop, and the thickened uterine lining is shed during the menstrual period.

The Thyroid Impact

No one knows exactly how the thyroid hormones influence a woman's monthly cycle, but in women with thyroid disease, the monthly menstrual cycle can be significantly altered or disrupted. A thyroid problem can also affect teenage girls. Girls who get their period very early—before the age of ten—may be suffering from an overactive thyroid. Those who are fifteen or older when they get their first period may have hypothyroidism.

In women who have hypothyroidism, it's not uncommon for their periods to become much heavier than before. The duration of their periods may also increase, or they may notice that their cycle has gotten shorter, and they're getting their periods more frequently.

According to one study, approximately 23 percent of women with hypothyroidism experience menstrual irregularities. Other estimates have found that the impact is significantly higher.

The problems are different in women who have hyperthyroidism. Women whose thyroids are overactive tend to experience lighter periods, less frequent periods, or even complete absence of their monthly cycles. Approximately 22 percent of hyperthyroid women have menstrual problems, though again, some estimates suggest the rate is much higher. The most common disturbances are defined as:

Amenorrhea

Amenorrhea is the medical term for the lack of menstrual periods. In women who have been menstruating, it is called secondary amenorrhea and defined by the absence of periods for more than three to six months. It is also diagnosed in girls who have not had their first periods by the age of sixteen and is called primary amenorrhea.

Oligomenorrhea

When a woman has fewer than six to eight menstrual periods in a year, she may be diagnosed with oligomenorrhea, or infrequent periods. While some women may celebrate the fact that their periods have become less frequent, diminished frequency is usually a sign of a potential medical problem such as thyroid disease.

Dysmenorrhea

In some women, hypothyroidism can cause painful menstrual periods, known as dysmenorrhea. Dysmenorrhea can also involve lower back pain, nausea, bowel problems, achiness in the lower extremities, and excessive bloating.

Menorrhagia

Extremely heavy or prolonged menstrual bleeding is called menorrhagia. Women with menorrhagia may need to change their sanitary pad every hour over the period of several hours.

Shortened Cycles

Some women with hypothyroidism will notice that their menstrual cycle shortens by a few days. They may also have bleeding that lasts longer.

Call the Doctor

It's not unusual for healthy women to sometimes skip a period, have a delayed period, or experience changes in the heaviness of their flow. But some signs warrant medical attention. You should call your doctor if you:

- Have periods that occur less than twenty-one days apart
- Have not had a period for more than three months
- Are experiencing greater pain with your periods
- Bleed heavily for more than seventy-two hours
- Have periods that routinely last more than a week
- Get your period at age eight or nine
- Do not get your period until age sixteen or older

When trying to determine the cause of your menstrual irregularities, your doctor should consider many factors, including your thyroid. He should ask you about your personal and family history; medications you are taking; recent stress; and changes in your diet, exercise, and weight. He should ask about other signs and symptoms. A problem with your hypothalamus or pituitary, for example, may be accompanied by headache or vision problems. Significant weight loss may be a sign of anorexia or bulimia. The presence of hot flashes may suggest the onset of menopause.

If hypothyroidism is at the root of your menstrual irregularities, proper treatment usually corrects the disturbance. But the key, again, is establishing the right dose, so that you are at the right TSH level. The same is true if you are experiencing hyperthyroidism—you must strive to be at your optimal TSH level. If you are at the right TSH level but are still experiencing menstrual problems, you may need to consult with an endocrinologist who specializes in reproductive disorders.

Imitators of Thyroid Disease

Many health conditions mimic aspects of thyroid disease, a fact that makes diagnosis one of the biggest hurdles to getting treatment. The constant fatigue may suggest depression. Weight gain may be a sign of metabolic syndrome. Anxiety may lead to a diagnosis of panic disorder. In this chapter, you'll take a look at some of the common conditions that may be confused with thyroid disease.

Depression

Everyone goes through an occasional bout of the blues, but for some people, these spells of sadness are actually depression, a serious mental illness that can cause tremendous pain and suffering. People with depression often stop enjoying events and activities that once were pleasurable. For some, just getting through each day can become a challenge. In severe cases, suicide can be the devastating consequence.

According to the National Institute of Mental Health, almost 19 million people in the United States suffer from a depressive illness in a given year—almost 10 percent of the population. Women are affected twice as often as men. Depression is also the leading cause of disability in the world, according to the World Health Organization.

It's easy to mistake hypothyroidism for depression. After all, depression can be a symptom of thyroid disease, usually hypothyroidism. And both conditions can bring on fatigue, memory problems, and trouble sleeping. They can also cause weight gain and inexplicable aches and pains. Take Mary Ann, who experienced severe depression before she was diagnosed with hypothyroidism:

> Mary Ann and her husband had been married for only a year when she sank into a deep funk. She cried all the time and never felt happy about anything in her life. Her depression was so severe that she considered leaving her husband, thinking she had married the wrong man and that maybe she was better off single. Fortunately, a doctor's visit quickly led to a diagnosis of hypothyroidism. Today, Mary Ann has three children and is happily married.

Many signs and symptoms of depression are subtle and easily blamed on stress, fatigue, and a hectic lifestyle. But as Mary Ann's story shows, depression may also suggest that you have an underactive thyroid.

Some experts argue that everyone with depression should be tested for thyroid disease. But many well-meaning doctors will simply prescribe an antidepressant without considering that a thyroid disorder may be at the root. If you suspect that your depression is linked to your thyroid, insist on a thyroid test, especially if you have a family or personal history of thyroid or autoimmune disease.

Diabetes and Insulin Resistance

Diabetes is an endocrine disorder that results when the body no longer produces enough of the hormone insulin or can't respond to the insulin it does produce. As a result, glucose cannot be converted into energy, and excess glucose is left to linger in the blood, wreaking havoc throughout the body.

Though type 1 diabetes causes the same problem, type 1 is actually an autoimmune disease that results when the pancreas stops producing insulin. Type 2 diabetes is the kind that develops slowly, often as the result of an unhealthy lifestyle and excess weight. Many people who develop diabetes start with a condition known as insulin resistance, also called prediabetes or metabolic syndrome.

Alert

Even if your blood sugar level is fine, you may still have metabolic syndrome, which is often a precursor to diabetes and heart disease. Men with metabolic syndrome have a waistline more than forty inches, and women, thirty-five inches. They may also have high blood pressure, high triglycerides, low HDL cholesterol, and high LDL cholesterol.

Diabetes affects an estimated 21 million people in the United States. The rise in the incidence of diabetes corresponds with a parallel increase in the numbers of people who are overweight and obese. And although it was once primarily a condition of the elderly, today diabetes occurs even in children and young adults. Many health experts blame the rise in diabetes on inactive lifestyles and poor diets.

For some people, the symptoms of insulin resistance and diabetes may seem remarkably similar to hypothyroidism. There's the excess weight, the fatigue, and an overall feeling of sluggishness. Some people with diabetes may actually lose weight as the body breaks down stores of fat and muscle for energy, which could be confused with hyperthyroidism. Diabetes also causes numbness and tingling, slow-healing cuts and infections, and weakness—all symptoms that smack of hypothyroidism.

But diabetes differs in that many people experience frequent urination and extreme thirst. Frequent bathroom trips are the result of the kidneys working overtime to rid the body of excess sugar. The extreme thirst occurs as the sugar soaks up water, causing dehydration of body cells. These are often the first signs of diabetes. To confirm whether you have diabetes, your doctor may perform one of several kinds of glucose tests.

Either way, people who have diabetes or hypothyroidism seem to be at greater risk for developing the other condition.

Polycystic Ovarian Syndrome (PCOS)

Difficulty getting pregnant. The absence of menstrual periods. Inexplicable weight gain. While these symptoms sound like those in thyroid disease, they could be PCOS.

No one knows exactly what causes PCOS, but some experts believe the problem has to do with the body's inability to respond appropriately to insulin, a hormone that helps the body convert glucose into energy. There may also be a genetic link since women with PCOS often have a mother or sister with it, too. The condition affects 5 to 10 percent of all women and is the most common reproductive problem in women of childbearing age.

PCOS occurs when the ovaries produce too much testosterone. Sometimes the overproduction of testosterone is a result of the pituitary gland making too much LH. It can also occur when there is insulin resistance in the body cells, which leads to an abundance of insulin in the bloodstream. Being overweight can cause a rise in insulin, which can trigger PCOS, but the condition is not limited to women who are overweight.

Every month or so, in healthy women, ten to twenty eggs start to mature, until a single mature egg is released from the ovaries, causing ovulation. PCOS occurs when the ovaries don't make enough hormones to cause the eggs to mature. Instead, the eggs grow and become cysts. These cysts produce testosterone, which suppresses menstruation and causes unwanted hair growth.

Essential

Women with PCOS often have cysts around the border of the ovary in a pattern often described as a string of pearls. These cysts are similar to ovarian cysts, which are larger and occur inside the ovary. Unlike ovarian cysts, however, which can burst and cause pain, the cysts in PCOS typically go unnoticed.

Both hypothyroidism and PCOS cause irregular menstrual periods, weight gain, high cholesterol, and high blood pressure. They can both cause fatigue, depression, and infertility. But unlike thyroid disease, PCOS may also cause acne; oily skin; and hair growth on the face, chest, and stomach.

Chronic Fatigue Immune Deficiency Syndrome (CFIDS)

Fatigue has become a part of our modern, harried lives. Every day, we juggle jobs, children, and chores on a cycle that leaves many of us exhausted.

But CFIDS, also called chronic fatigue syndrome (CFS), is much more than ordinary tiredness. With CFIDS, the fatigue is strong, persistent, and debilitating, typically making you too weak to perform everyday tasks and activities. The exhaustion typically persists for no apparent reason. You're tired even when you have little to do or even after a good night's rest.

According to estimates by the Centers for Disease Control and Prevention, approximately 500,000 Americans suffer from CFIDS, the vast majority women. In the 1980s, CFIDS was called the yuppie flu because most sufferers were well-educated, middle- to upper-class women in their thirties and forties. Experts used to believe that CFIDS was the result of the Epstein-Barr virus, the same virus that causes mononucleosis. This notion has since been dismissed, but the cause of CFIDS remains a mystery. What we do know is that CFIDS can afflict people of any age, race, or socioeconomic status.

A diagnosis for CFIDS is usually made only after other medical conditions are ruled out. But CFIDS can coexist with other disorders such as depression. It can also resemble other illnesses, including hypothyroidism. Dr. Friedman thinks that most patients who have been diagnosed with CFIDS really have an undiagnosed endocrine problem.

⌐, Essential

> As of now, there is no cure for CFIDS. Instead, treatment aims to relieve the symptoms; for example, sleep remedies for insomnia, or antidepressants for depression. Those with CFIDS generally do benefit from lifestyle changes such as getting more exercise, eating well, and reducing stress.

Many symptoms of CFIDS may be confused with those of thyroid disease. People with CFIDS are, of course, tired, but they're also achy and having problems with memory. They may have headaches, joint aches, and muscle pain. Some people with CFIDS may experience weight loss, which may call to mind hyperthyroidism, especially if it's accompanied by a rapid pulse and problems sleeping, both symptoms of CFIDS.

CFIDS may cause a sore throat and tender lymph nodes. For someone who has trouble distinguishing a sore throat from thyroid pain, these symptoms may be incorrectly described to a doctor. But unlike thyroid disease, CFIDS cannot be detected in the blood. Instead, doctors must rely on patient reports of specific symptoms.

Fibromyalgia

Until recent years, many people questioned the existence of fibromyalgia. But most experts now agree that fibromyalgia is a distinct medical condition characterized by widespread pain, sleep problems, tender points around the body, and a host of other symptoms that range from irritable bowel syndrome to depression. Still, fibromyalgia is a baffling condition, one that is hard to diagnose and difficult to treat.

According to the National Institutes of Arthritis, Musculoskeletal, and Skin Diseases, fibromyalgia affects 3 to 6 million people in the United States, which means one in fifty Americans has this condition. The majority of sufferers are women, but the condition also occurs in men and children of all ages and races. Although the condition starts at a younger age, experts estimate that more than 7 percent of women between the ages of sixty and seventy-nine have fibromyalgia.

The symptoms of fibromyalgia vary drastically from one patient to another, but almost everyone experiences a degree of pain and fatigue. Other common problems include memory problems, trouble concentrating, painful menstrual periods, headaches, and intolerance for cold temperatures.

But people with fibromyalgia may also experience other problems that do not occur in hypothyroidism. For instance, fibro sufferers often suffer from restless legs syndrome, an irresistible urge to move your legs during sleep as the result of abnormal sensations. They may also have temporomandibular joint disorder, numbness and tingling in the extremities, and morning stiffness.

Diagnosing fibromyalgia is tricky. Like CFIDS, there are no blood tests or X-rays that confirm fibromyalgia, so doctors are left to rely only on self-reported symptoms. Doctors may also do palpation tests on tender points. Many times, diagnosis is made after other conditions—such as hypothyroidism—are ruled out. If you're having these symptoms, ask your doctor to check your thyroid.

Lupus

Lupus is an autoimmune disorder that occurs when the body's immune system attacks its own cells and tissues, especially the skin, joints, blood, and kidneys. No one knows what causes the immune system to go awry, but in lupus, this autoimmune attack produces a host of symptoms, which vary widely in types and intensity from one patient to the next.

Experts estimate there are 500,000 to 1.5 million Americans who have been diagnosed with lupus. Only about 10 percent of people with the condition have a parent or sibling with the illness, and only about 5 percent of children born to parents with lupus eventually develop it. That's why environmental factors such as stress, illness, and ultraviolet light are believed to play a role in the onset of lupus.

And because the disease afflicts women more than men, some experts suspect that hormones play a role.

Fact

There are actually three types of lupus: systemic lupus erythematosus (SLE), discoid, and drug-induced. SLE is the most severe kind, the type most people have, and the kind that can affect various organs and body systems. Discoid affects only the skin. Drug-induced lupus results from taking certain drugs, such as hydralazine, which is used to treat high blood pressure, and procainamide, which is used to treat irregular heart rhythms.

Almost everyone who has lupus experiences extreme fatigue, which is one reason why it may sometimes be confused with hypothyroidism. People with lupus may also suffer from joint pain, a low-grade fever, anemia, and a rash. They may also have hair loss, kidney problems, and Raynaud's phenomenon, in which the fingers turn white in reaction to cold temperatures. But many times, the symptoms of lupus are vague, and they often come and go, making it hard to figure out exactly what is going on.

Like thyroid disease, diagnosing lupus involves blood tests. The presence of certain autoantibodies is often a telltale sign that you have lupus and not a thyroid problem.

However, having lupus does not mean that you do not also have a thyroid problem. In fact, having lupus raises your risk for other autoimmune conditions such as Hashimoto's disease and Graves' disease. That's why you should also ask your doctor to do a thyroid test. Treating a thyroid problem can lessen the symptoms caused by lupus.

Cushing's Syndrome

In healthy people, the hormone cortisol plays a vital role in dealing with stress, prepping the body to fight or flee from a tough situation.

Our ancestors relied on it to escape wild animals; we get a surge of it whenever we are facing a deadline, fighting with our spouse, or dealing with rush-hour traffic. In people who have prolonged exposure to excess amounts of cortisol, the result is sometimes Cushing's syndrome, a rare disease that affects adults between the ages of twenty and fifty, mainly women.

People develop Cushing's for several reasons. The condition may occur in people who have taken steroids such as prednisone for the long-term treatment of asthma, lupus, or rheumatoid arthritis. In others, Cushing's is caused by the body's making too much cortisol. Tumors or illnesses affecting the pituitary or adrenals can wreak havoc on the adrenal gland's production of cortisol. In extremely rare cases, Cushing's is an inherited disorder that causes a tendency for tumors on one or more of the endocrine glands.

Some people may have a milder form of the disease called pseudo-Cushing's, in which the patient has elevated cortisol as in Cushing's but has fewer signs and symptoms than someone with full-blown Cushing's.

Question

Can too much stress cause Cushing's?
No, but stress can cause a host of health problems—depression, insomnia, anxiety, and weight gain—that lead to other health problems such as heart disease. On its own, stress doesn't lead to full-blown Cushing's syndrome—or else we'd have a Cushing's epidemic.

Pseudo-Cushing's is not caused by a tumor, but may be the result of myriad health problems, including depression, alcoholism, surgery-related stress, severe illness, and poorly controlled diabetes. Pseudo-Cushing's doesn't cause the progressive problems associated with Cushing's, such as weakening bones, fractures, and thinning of the skin. But when the symptoms are mild and vague, it is easy to confuse pseudo-Cushing's with a thyroid disorder.

Though symptoms vary, some cases of Cushing's disease do bear a resemblance to hypothyroidism. Many people may notice weight gain, especially in the upper body, and a rounding and reddening of the face. The skin may be fragile and thin, and there may be loss of muscle strength, high blood pressure, and high blood sugar. Patients may also develop purplish pink stretch marks on the arms, abdomen, thighs, buttocks, and breasts. Most people are severely fatigued and will experience irritability, anxiety, and depression.

Women with Cushing's may have menstrual irregularities and excess hair growth. Men may experience low libido and have problems with erections. Children with Cushing's may become obese and experience a slowdown in growth rate.

Diagnosing Cushing's can be difficult and involves an array of tests such as urine samples, CT scans, and MRIs. You will also need to undergo tests that measure levels of different hormones that affect the secretion of cortisol.

Panic Disorder

A rapid heartbeat. Nervousness. Trouble breathing. All these symptoms may suggest hyperthyroidism, but they can just as easily be pointing to an anxiety problem known as panic disorder. It's not uncommon at all for people with hyperthyroidism to be initially misdiagnosed as having panic disorder.

Panic disorder is a type of anxiety disorder. People with anxiety are consumed with worry. Their worrying is disproportionate to the actual event and is frequently accompanied by physical problems such as headaches, fatigue, irritability, sleep difficulty, and muscle tension.

No one knows the exact cause of panic disorder, but the condition often develops after a stressful event. Panic disorder affects about 2.4 million Americans between ages eighteen and fifty-four. It often first strikes in young adulthood before age twenty-four and is more common in women than men.

People who have panic disorder suffer from unexpected and repeated episodes of intense fear known as panic attacks. Symptoms include heart palpitations, shortness of breath, chest pain, tingling, dizziness, or abdominal pain. They may feel a sense of impending doom as the panic attack intensifies. Taking these facts into account, it's easy to see why hyperthyroidism is confused with panic disorder. The two conditions have similar symptoms, and both emerge in young adulthood. But if you have a family or personal history of thyroid disease, you might want to ask for a thyroid test before getting officially diagnosed with panic disorder. Hyperthyroidism can also exacerbate panic disorder.

 Fact

According to the American Psychological Association, panic disorder is tough to diagnose. People sometimes visit ten or more doctors before getting properly diagnosed, and one in four people with this condition is never diagnosed.

Sleep Apnea

Approximately 18 million people in the United States have sleep apnea, a potentially serious sleep disorder that occurs when you actually stop breathing for ten to thirty seconds at a time while you're asleep. These brief spells can occur numerous times a night, causing disruptions in breathing that may awaken you from sound sleep and prevent a good night's rest. During sleep, the person with sleep apnea may frequently snore, pause, and gasp. During the day, the person with sleep apnea is very tired. Some people, however, are unaware they have sleep apnea until a family member tells them of these nightly disturbances.

Sleep apnea may be obstructive, central, or mixed. With obstructive sleep apnea, the blockage is caused by the collapse of soft tissue in the rear of the throat during sleep. In central sleep apnea, the airway is open, but the brain fails to signal the muscles to breathe. Mixed sleep apnea is a combination of the two. Sleep apnea can occur in people of all ages, but your risk rises if you're overweight, over the age of forty, and male.

Essential

Studies show that people who have sleep apnea are especially vulnerable to job performance difficulties and motor vehicle crashes. If you suspect you have sleep apnea, take extra precautions while driving or operating heavy machinery.

Over time, sleep apnea can cause weight gain, fatigue, memory problems, and headaches. Men have trouble with erections, and women may have high blood pressure, memory problems, weight gain, and headaches. Eventually, some people develop depression.

As you know, many of these symptoms are remarkably similar to those you experience with hypothyroidism. And if you don't know that you're snoring at night, you may not even suspect sleep apnea as the cause of your symptoms. But if a thyroid test shows that your thyroid hormone levels are normal, you should ask your doctor for an evaluation for sleep apnea.

The evaluation is called a sleep study, or polysomnography, and usually involves an overnight stay in a sleep clinic. During the night, various monitors and recording equipment will be used to measure your heart rate, eye movements, muscle movements, oral and nasal airflow, and blood-oxygen levels. These measures will determine the severity of your sleep apnea and decide your course of treatment.

Menopause

Menopause is not a disease or a medical condition. It's a natural biological process, a life change—often called The Change—that signals the end of a woman's reproductive years. It can also be an incredibly difficult time for some women, who experience numerous physical symptoms, including the infamous hot flashes.

Although most people associate menopause with your fifties, menopause actually starts to occur in your late thirties and forties, when periods start to become increasingly irregular. This irregularity is caused by a natural decline in the body's production of estrogen and progesterone. Eventually, when you don't have a period for twelve consecutive months, you are said to have reached menopause. The majority of women will experience menopause between the ages of forty-five and fifty-five.

Some women glide through menopause without any symptoms at all, just the gradual cessation of their periods. But other women will notice several symptoms, including:

- Weight gain, especially in the abdominal area
- Memory and concentration problems
- Spotting between periods
- Mood swings and irritability
- Muscle aches and pains
- Hot flashes in which you feel warm in the chest and face
- Dryness in the vagina
- Low libido

As you can see, some of these symptoms resemble those of hypothyroidism, especially weight gain and memory and concentration problems. Others such as hot flashes and muscle aches and pains may suggest hyperthyroidism. Depending on when these symptoms first occur, you may be more apt to suspect the onset of menopause than a thyroid problem.

But if you do experience these symptoms, it's important to have a thyroid test. While it's true that you may be experiencing menopause, you may also be dealing with a simultaneous thyroid disorder. Women who have a thyroid disease in menopause are at greater risk for heart disease than those without thyroid disease. They're also at increased risk for osteoporosis.

Growth Hormone (GH) Deficiency

To achieve adult height, everyone needs GH. But some people are born with inadequate amounts of GH—called congenital growth hormone deficiency—and others may acquire the problem later on.

A deficit in GH in children has been recognized for decades, in large part because the problem is so apparent. Children without enough GH simply don't grow and develop normally. Growth is significantly slowed, and the child often slips to the lower percentages on height and weight charts. Your child may also have delayed puberty.

But the condition was largely unrecognized in adults until the 1990s. That's when experts realized that GH affected virtually every type of body tissue. Experts also learned that a deficit in GH is associated with higher mortality.

GH deficiency most often develops as a result of a problem with the pituitary gland, caused by a tumor or surgery or radiation to treat that tumor. When something goes wrong with the pituitary gland, GH is one of the first hormones to be affected.

Diagnosing GH deficiency involves the use of stimulation testing. One test is called an insulin-tolerance test, in which low blood glucose is achieved by insulin administration. Blood is drawn to measure GH. Another test more widely used is called an Arginine-GHRH test, in which arginine, an amino acid, and GH-releasing hormone are injected into the body. Blood measurements are then done to see how much GH is released.

Adults without enough GH tend to experience a decrease in muscle, an increase in fat, and a reduction in exercise capacity. Some people with GH deficiency will experience sleep problems, fatigue, and depression. Because some of these symptoms are the same as those in hypothyroidism, the two conditions can easily be mistaken for one another.

CHAPTER 14

Pregnancy and Your Thyroid

Getting pregnant is an incredibly exciting event that indicates big life changes to come. Of course, pregnancy can also have some profound effects on your body. And if you have thyroid disease, pregnancy can become a bit more complicated. In this chapter, you'll take a look at the impact thyroid disease has on fertility, pregnancy, and postpartum, including special concerns for the mom-to-be and her baby.

The Thyroid in Pregnancy

During pregnancy, every part of your body is affected. Your blood flow increases. Your lungs work harder. Even your hair grows faster. So it should come as no surprise that the thyroid gland is affected, too.

In pregnancy, two hormones in particular can affect the thyroid: human chorionic gonadotropin (HCG) and estrogen. HCG is a hormone produced early on in pregnancy by the placenta. In fact, most pregnancy tests work by detecting the presence of HCG. During pregnancy, HCG behaves similarly to TSH and can sometimes cause the thyroid gland to become slightly larger. Usually, this enlargement isn't significant and is not even noticeable except on ultrasound. The HCG can also sometimes cause TSH levels to dip in the first trimester, so at that time, your thyroid tests will show a slightly low TSH and slightly elevated T4. Your dose of thyroid hormone, however, is unlikely to change.

Estrogen goes up in the second and third trimesters and causes an increase in TBG, the protein that binds thyroid hormone. When TBG goes up, the amount of total T4 and T3 goes up. The increase in total T4 and T3 usually does not affect levels of free T4 and T3, which are the hormones actually available to your body cells.

For patients without hypothyroidism, the body compensates and no treatment is needed. The mother's blood gets diluted as it goes to the placenta and the baby. However, extra TBG binds to levothyroxine in patients who take thyroid hormone replacement. That's why women on thyroid hormone replacement typically need higher doses during the second half of pregnancy.

For a pregnancy to occur and to be healthy, it's important to maintain normal levels of TSH, free T4, and free T3. For healthy women, this comes naturally, without extra effort. But if you have a thyroid disorder, you may need extra medical intervention to achieve and maintain this healthy state of affairs.

When You're Trying to Conceive

Few things in life are more exciting than the prospect of having a baby. The good news is that having thyroid disease does not necessarily prevent you from having a child. In fact, most women who have thyroid disease conceive with little effort and have perfectly healthy pregnancies and babies.

Even women who have a history of thyroid cancer can still have a perfectly healthy pregnancy and normal baby. There is no evidence to show that thyroid cancer or its treatments causes birth defects or difficulties with pregnancy. The only caveat comes into play if you've had RAI treatment, which simply means you might need to wait a few months before conceiving. The exact amount of time depends on your doctor.

Alert

Women with subclinical hypothyroidism may have no problem getting pregnant. But they are generally at higher risk for miscarriage, stillbirth, and premature birth. Any woman with repeated miscarriages and problems carrying a baby to term should consider having her thyroid tested.

Other women with thyroid disease, however, wrestle with serious problems, especially if the condition goes undetected and untreated. For starters, you may not be able to even get pregnant. Others may get pregnant, but then suffer problems such as miscarriage, pre-eclampsia, and premature labor and delivery. And if you carry the baby to term, the baby may inherit your thyroid condition and experience problems with growth and development. Severe cases may lead to mental retardation and birth defects. (See Chapter 16 for more on children and thyroid disease.)

In reality, those are the exceptions. Plenty of women have battled thyroid disease and gone on to have perfectly healthy babies. The key is making sure that you are routinely monitored and that your condition is under control before you get pregnant.

As soon as you learn you're pregnant, it's important to tell your obstetrician-gynecologist if you've ever had, or currently have, a thyroid problem. You should also tell your doctor if you have a family history of thyroid problems.

You should also let your endocrinologist know about your plans to conceive, so that he will keep an eye on your TSH levels and make sure you're getting enough medication to keep your disease in check. Making the effort to take precautions will help ensure that you have a healthy pregnancy—and a healthy baby.

Before Getting Pregnant

Healthy women take it for granted that their thyroid glands are churning out the right amount of thyroid hormone. But if you're contemplating pregnancy and have hypo- or hyperthyroidism, it's essential to make sure you have the proper amount of thyroid hormone. That means getting the disease under control *before* you get pregnant.

Even if you don't have thyroid disease right now, you may want to have your thyroid checked if you have a family or personal history of thyroid disease. You may also want to check your thyroid if you have a family or personal history of conditions associated with thyroid problems such as type 1 diabetes, vitiligo, or celiac disease.

If your TSH test shows that you are hypo- or hyperthyroid, make sure to get treated and to follow up with your doctor to see if your TSH becomes normal. (We discuss both conditions and their treatments in detail in Chapters 4 through 9.)

You should also talk to your doctor about the best time for you and your partner to start trying to get pregnant. Different doctors will have different opinions about the ideal TSH for conceiving. But ideally, you should at least be close to having healthy thyroid function before you try to get pregnant.

Infertility

You've gotten the green light, but months later, you're still not pregnant. For some women with thyroid disease, getting pregnant may be the biggest challenge of all. Many factors can make a couple infertile. Sexually transmitted diseases, cigarette smoking, and advancing age can all make it harder for a couple to conceive. Thyroid disease can also make conception difficult.

Women who have thyroid disease sometimes develop menstrual irregularities for numerous reasons. These problems include:

- Lack of ovulation, so there is no egg released for conception to occur. This may occur in both hypo- and hyperthyroidism.

- PCOS, a condition that causes cysts on the ovaries and inhibits pregnancy. PCOS is more common in women with hypothyroidism.
- Irregular menstrual cycles that make pregnancy difficult. Menstruation can be affected by both hypo- and hyperthyroidism.
- Excess prolactin, a hormone released by the pituitary gland that stimulates milk production after delivery and that may inhibit ovulation. This problem may occur in women with severe hypothyroidism.

In most cases, proper treatment of the underlying thyroid disease will resolve these problems. But if fertility is still a challenge, you or your partner may have another health problem that warrants medical attention.

Question

How do I know if I'm ovulating?
An ovulation predictor kit is your best bet. The stick turns color the day before you ovulate in response to an increase in luteinizing hormone (LH), the hormone that triggers ovulation. You can also try charting basal body temperature first thing in the morning over a few months to figure out when you ovulate. An increase in body temperature usually indicates you're ovulating.

Miscarriages

Women who have hyperthyroidism may have a hard time staying pregnant. Hyperthyroidism increases your risk for miscarriage, which is the premature loss of a pregnancy. Women who have repeated miscarriages and have signs or symptoms of hyperthyroidism should definitely have their thyroid function checked. Again, treatment for the thyroid disease can usually resolve the difficulties unless there is another underlying problem.

Thyroid Disease During Pregnancy

After months of trying, you're delighted to learn that you're pregnant. For most women with thyroid disease that's well controlled, these blissful months will progress uneventfully. But having thyroid disease does raise your risk for certain complications such as preeclampsia. That usually means more trips to the doctor's office, more blood tests, and, potentially, adjustments to your thyroid medications.

Of course, pregnancy affects different women differently. For some women who already have Hashimoto's or Graves' disease, being pregnant can sometimes put the disease into a welcome remission. Pregnancy has a naturally calming effect on the immune system, which prevents the mom from rejecting the fetal tissue. As a result, autoimmune conditions often seem to take a breather, and you wind up feeling better during pregnancy.

Essential

Pregnant women have higher requirements for iodine than women who are not. According to the Institute of Medicine, pregnant women need 220 mcg of iodine a day instead of the 150 mcg a day normally suggested for adolescents and adults. This amount is easily obtained in your diet and in your prenatal vitamin.

But in some cases, pregnancy seems to trigger the onset of thyroid disease. This situation can be challenging. It isn't easy to spot thyroid disease in a pregnant woman. Many of the symptoms of both hypo- and hyperthyroidism resemble those you see in pregnancy. Fatigue, mood swings, and constipation are all common in hypothyroidism and pregnancy. And like pregnant women, those who have hyperthyroidism may experience a faster pulse, nervousness, and greater sensitivity to warmth and heat.

Usually, it takes a skilled physician to distinguish the normal symptoms of pregnancy from those of thyroid disease—one who has the smarts to order a blood test for TSH. But it also requires that the patient realize that what she's feeling is more than just pregnancy-related problems and to report these symptoms to the doctor. It also helps to know your family history for autoimmune and thyroid diseases. Jane, for example, had no idea of her family history of thyroid disease, and began her battle with thyroid disease during pregnancy.

For starters, Jane had a hard time getting pregnant. When she finally did, she started feeling anxious and developed a rapid heartbeat, which she attributed to her pregnancy. After a difficult labor, Jane sank into a postpartum depression that she couldn't seem to shake, even after a few years. Tests revealed that she had Hashimoto's disease, and she was given Synthroid. She later learned that her mother, along with several aunts, all had Hashimoto's disease.

If you do develop a thyroid disorder in pregnancy, it's important to get diagnosed and treated as soon as possible. Prompt treatment will help ensure that the disease does not affect the developing fetus.

Hypothyroidism

Most cases of hypothyroidism in pregnancy are the result of Hashimoto's disease. In some cases, a woman may develop hypothyroidism because the dosage of thyroid hormone replacement became inadequate in pregnancy. Women can also develop hypothyroidism from overtreatment with antithyroid medications for hyperthyroidism.

Untreated hypothyroidism has serious consequences for both mother and baby. A mother may be at risk for:

- Anemia
- Muscle weakness

- Pre-eclampsia, high blood pressure and protein in the urine that can lead to kidney damage
- Heart failure
- Problems with the placenta
- Postpartum bleeding

A baby whose mother has untreated hypothyroidism may be at risk for:

- Low birth weight
- Congenital hypothyroidism
- Impaired brain development
- Developmental abnormalities
- Learning problems
- Mental retardation

Treating Hypothyroidism in Pregnancy

Fortunately, treatment for hypothyroidism is relatively easy. Like anyone with hypothyroidism, pregnant women need thyroid hormone replacement, which, in the right dose, is perfectly safe to take in pregnancy. Establishing the right dose is critical, and you will need frequent testing to determine if your thyroid hormone levels are healthy.

Pre-existing Hypothyroidism

In women who already have hypothyroidism, it's important to have your thyroid tested as soon as you find out you're pregnant. Don't let your doctor delay your appointment, and take steps to clear your schedule so that your doctor's visit is a top priority.

Your dose of levothyroxine can increase with pregnancy, especially in the second half of pregnancy, often by 25 to 50 percent. In some cases, it may even double. Your doctor should do regular tests of thyroid function throughout your pregnancy to ensure that your TSH levels remain normal, and if a change in your dosage becomes necessary, more frequent testing may be needed.

Alert

Don't take your thyroid hormone at the same time you take your prenatal vitamins. The American Thyroid Association (ATA) recommends separating the two drugs by two to three hours. Prenatal vitamins contain iron, which can inhibit absorption of thyroid hormone.

Careful monitoring of your thyroid is essential throughout your pregnancy, not only for you, but for your developing baby, who relies on you to supply her with enough thyroid hormone. Take your medicine diligently, keep all your doctor appointments, and follow through on changes in the dosage of your medication.

Hyperthyroidism

As in the general population, the most common cause of hyperthyroidism in pregnancy is Graves' disease. But diagnosing hyperthyroidism can be tricky. Pregnant women cannot have an RAIU and scan because the radioactivity could potentially affect the baby's developing thyroid gland.

But untreated and active Graves' disease poses serious risks to both the mother and the baby. In the mother, the risks include:

- Pre-eclampsia, high blood pressure and protein in the urine that can lead to kidney damage
- Premature labor
- Thyroid storm

In the baby, a mother's active Graves' disease can raise the risk for several problems, including:

- Fetal tachycardia (rapid heartbeat)
- Low birth weight
- Prematurity

- Stillbirth
- Neonatal hyperthyroidism
- Goiter

Treating Hyperthyroidism in Pregnancy

Unless you have a mild case of hyperthyroidism that is causing no symptoms, not treating hyperthyroidism is simply not an option. The risks associated with untreated hyperthyroidism are high and outweigh any risks associated with the use of treatment. Still, treatment for this condition can be more complicated during pregnancy since your options are more limited.

⌐ Essential

Many moms experience morning sickness in their first trimester. But if it lingers, you may be suffering from higher than normal levels of HCG, which can cause severe morning sickness and trigger the overproduction of thyroid hormone, a condition known as transient hyperthyroidism. To treat this condition, the pregnant mom is usually given a beta-blocker for a few weeks.

Like any case of hyperthyroidism, the goal of treatment is to lower the amount of thyroid hormone. Most often, the therapy of choice is PTU, which is considered a safer option in pregnancy than the other antithyroid drug, methimazole (Tapazole).

Most doctors will aim to get your free T4 and free T3 levels into the high-normal range on the lowest possible dose of PTU. But establishing the right dose can be tough. Too much PTU can affect the baby and cause hypothyroidism and goiter. It can also trigger hypothyroidism in the mother.

And yet, you need enough antithyroid medication to reduce the amount of thyroid hormone circulating in the mom. That's why treatment always involves routine monitoring to make sure TSH and thyroid hormone levels are close to normal. Given the choice, most doctors would prefer pregnant patients to be slightly hyperthyroid rather than slightly hypothyroid. If you're hypothyroid, the risk to your baby is greater.

If a pregnant woman is allergic to or has a reaction to PTU, she may be given methimazole instead. If neither drug can be tolerated, you may require surgery to remove the overactive thyroid. Because any kind of surgery comes with inherent risks, it is not commonly done in pregnant women. RAI treatment (and scans) is never used in pregnant women because the radioactivity can destroy the baby's developing thyroid and cause permanent hypothyroidism.

To combat the symptoms of hyperthyroidism, your doctor may prescribe a beta-blocker such as atenolol. But these drugs are generally used with caution. Taken in excess, they can impair fetal growth and cause low birth weight.

Hyperthyroidism and Your Baby

Even if you're successfully treated for hyperthyroidism, and you take the smallest dose of medication possible, your developing baby is still at risk for a condition called neonatal thyrotoxicosis, which is basically hyperthyroidism. This condition is most likely to occur in women whose hyperthyroidism is caused by Graves' disease.

As you might recall, Graves' disease is accompanied by the presence of TSIs. Antithyroid medications and surgery do not destroy TSIs, which continue to linger in your blood and can transfer to your baby. In very rare cases, a developing baby may develop thyrotoxicosis while in utero. This condition tends to occur in women with Graves' disease who have very high levels of TSI. Intrauterine thyrotoxicosis can cause fetal tachycardia, failure to grow, advanced aging of the bones, and occasionally fetal death. Babies whose moms have elevated TSI should be carefully monitored before and after delivery.

〔. Essential

> Some developing babies whose mothers are taking PTU (or methimazole) may also develop hypothyroidism, especially if the dose is too high. An astute obstetrician may perform an ultrasound to determine if the fetus has a goiter. In that case, your dose may be reduced.

Although the numbers of babies of mothers with Graves' disease who become hyperthyroid is small, it's essential to detect it early since the condition is potentially fatal. For that reason, if you have hyperthyroidism, you should have your baby's thyroid tested at birth and soon after with your pediatrician.

Other Thyroid Problems

Pregnancy does not spare you from developing other thyroid problems such as nodules, goiters, and cancer. For more specific information about these conditions, see Chapters 10 and 11. But pregnancy does make diagnosis and treatment much more challenging. For instance, while you can still have an FNA on a nodule, you should not have an RAIU and scan while you are pregnant.

In some cases, your doctor may recommend a wait-and-see approach to see if your thyroid problem worsens, with the hopes of delaying treatment such as surgery until after you've delivered. In other cases, however, waiting is not an option. Finding a cancerous nodule that is large and painful, for instance, may require immediate surgery regardless of your pregnancy. Each case must be handled individually.

To ensure the best possible outcome, seek out an endocrinologist and/or surgeon who has had training, education, and experience in dealing with these special circumstances. Travel the distance if you must to locate a physician in a major metropolitan hospital if you don't have one nearby. The health and well-being of you and your unborn child are at stake, and finding the best care is essential.

Postpartum Thyroid Troubles

After having your baby, your thyroid naturally goes through another period of adjustment. Approximately 10 percent of all women will have some sort of postpartum thyroid problem, including the onset of an autoimmune thyroid disease or postpartum thyroiditis.

During this time, the immune system is readjusting and returning to its normal state. As you probably recall, the immune system is suppressed during pregnancy to ensure that the mother's body doesn't reject the fetal tissue. In the postpartum period, this process reverses itself, and the immune system gradually resumes normal activity.

As a result, women who have Hashimoto's or Graves' disease may notice a resurgence of their symptoms or show a change in their TSH levels. Those who had increased their dose of levothyroxine for Hashimoto's disease, for instance, can often go back to their lower prepregnancy dose. Women with Graves' disease may notice a worsening of symptoms and need to increase their dose of antithyroid medication.

The postpartum period is also ripe for the onset of an autoimmune disease, such as Hashimoto's or Graves' disease. Women who develop these conditions after delivering a baby will undergo the same diagnostic tests and have the same treatment options as anyone else. For more information, see Chapters 6 and 9. But women who are nursing should not be given radioactive iodine treatments.

Postpartum Thyroiditis

Many women go through a difficult time after having their babies. They're tired from nightly awakenings and feedings. They may have mood swings and bouts of unexplained sadness and crying. They may also have anxiety, insomnia, and fatigue—all common to new moms.

But for some women, the symptoms are related to a condition called postpartum thyroiditis, in which the thyroid gland becomes inflamed. Women with a personal or family history of autoimmune disease are at higher risk for postpartum thyroiditis, as are those whose mothers had this condition.

Essential

In rare circumstances, severe blood loss during childbirth can cause a condition called Sheehan's syndrome, or postpartum hypopituitarism. The condition causes a reduction in hormones produced by the pituitary, including TSH, and can lead to hypothyroidism. In Sheehan's syndrome, you may also have a sudden drop in the stress hormone, cortisol, which can produce an adrenal emergency.

Postpartum thyroiditis often lasts six to nine months, then disappears on its own. In most cases, the condition begins two to three months after delivery and follows a similar pattern. The thyroid is initially overactive for a month or two, when the inflamed gland starts leaking excess thyroid hormone into the bloodstream. After that, as the hormone dissipates, it becomes underactive for a few months, before becoming normal again. The condition is diagnosed with a TSH test and the patient's self-reported symptoms.

It isn't always easy to detect postpartum thyroiditis. Most women attribute the symptoms to the normal exhaustion that comes with tending to a new baby and to the natural shifts in hormone. But some experts suspect that postpartum thyroiditis is the culprit behind postpartum depression, a condition in which women become clinically depressed after giving birth. That would make postpartum thyroiditis considerably more common than believed.

As with most thyroid disease, the severity of postpartum thyroiditis can vary widely. In some cases, the symptoms are mild and barely even noticed, in which case treatment is a matter of waiting it out. But in other cases, the symptoms may be more pronounced. You may feel anxious and nervous, and you may have trouble breathing. Or you may feel overly tired, sluggish, and depressed.

Women who do have more disturbing symptoms might be prescribed beta-blockers to tame their hyperthyroidism. They may also require an antithyroid medication such as PTU (see below about nursing considerations). If the condition is detected in its hypothyroid stage, you may be given thyroid hormone replacement. Some women with postpartum thyroiditis go on to develop permanent hypothyroidism.

In any case, if you do develop postpartum thyroiditis, be on the lookout for future thyroid problems. Women who have postpartum thyroiditis are more likely to develop thyroid disease, and are more likely to have postpartum thyroiditis with future pregnancies.

Nursing Concerns

Breastfed babies reap many benefits from their moms, and it goes well beyond the vitamins and minerals found in breast milk. Nursing infants also get brain-enhancing fatty acids and immune system boosters that can protect them from illness. And according to the American Academy of Pediatrics, babies who are breastfed exclusively for six months are less likely to have ear infections, respiratory illnesses, and diarrhea.

 Fact

Breastfeeding moms may benefit from nursing their babies, too. Studies show that women who breastfeed may have a lower risk of breast and ovarian cancer, and a decreased risk of hip fractures and osteoporosis.

But nursing moms with thyroid disease may wonder whether the drugs they take will affect their babies, too. The answer depends largely on the medicine you need, but also on the amount you take and whom you ask.

If you have hypothyroidism, thyroid hormone replacement drugs are generally fine, so long as you're on the correct dosage. Only small amounts of these drugs get into the breast milk. Too much thyroid hormone, on the other hand, can affect the baby, who is then at risk for hyperthyroidism, just as you are. So if you are taking thyroid hormones, you'll need routine TSH tests to make sure you're getting just the right dosage.

Treatments for hyperthyroidism are much more controversial. For starters, you cannot receive RAI treatments or undergo RAI scans if you are nursing. The RAI collects in breast milk and can be transferred to the baby, whose thyroid gland would take up the iodine. If you absolutely need to have RAI treatment—the Graves' disease has become severe, for instance—you'll be asked to stop nursing or told to delay the RAI until you're finished nursing.

For nursing moms, antithyroid drugs are usually a better choice. PTU is generally the preferred treatment because less of it seeps into breast milk than methimazole. Taking as low a dose as possible is best, if you nurse. One study done in Japan found that women can safely take PTU while breastfeeding, so long as the dose is 750 mg or less per day.

Nonetheless, doctors worry about the impact of PTU on nursing infants. According to a study in the journal *Pediatrics*, 44 percent of endocrinologists discourage breastfeeding while taking PTU. In the end, the decision to nurse and the need for medication rests with you and your physician.

The Battle with Weight

CHAPTER 15

You've tried everything to lose that extra weight. You've cut out desserts, made daily visits to the gym, and given up snacking in front of the TV at night. Still, those pounds refuse to budge. Now, you wonder, could it be a thyroid problem? Turns out, your thyroid just might be the bad guy. In this chapter, you'll learn how your thyroid affects your weight and what you can do about it.

How Your Thyroid Affects Weight

Anyone who has ever tried to lose weight knows the frustration. The endless dieting. The attempts to exercise. The ups and downs on the scale. When at long last your doctor figures out you have a thyroid problem, you pin your hopes on the thyroid hormone replacement drug, only to find, months later, that you're still embroiled in a battle with your weight.

Or perhaps you're part of the minority who has the opposite problem. No matter how much you eat, you can't seem to gain weight. You try eating more frequently. You try to eat more high-calorie foods. You indulge in desserts, snacks, and anything you want. Still, you remain thin as a rail and forever fighting off colds, flus, and other infections.

In both cases, the problem could have something to do with your thyroid. An underactive thyroid tells the body to slow down and harness its energy stores, causing an increase in appetite and an overall reduction in your metabolism. An overactive thyroid speeds everything up, so that cell activity is accelerated, causing energy in your body to be burned more quickly. (This chapter focuses on losing weight since that is the more common problem.)

Some people, like Beth, encounter weight changes on both ends of the spectrum.

Early on, Beth noticed she was losing weight, and had headaches, exhaustion, and a rapid heartbeat. A doctor uncovered her hyperthyroidism and suggested RAI treatment. Before the treatment, he encouraged her to eat whatever she wanted, and still, she lost 10 percent of her body weight. But after the RAI, her doctor waited six weeks before starting her on Synthroid. All the weight she lost came back until she got on Synthroid. Gradually, she lost the extra weight.

The thyroid gland plays a major role in body weight because it regulates your basal metabolic rate (BMR). That's the rate at which your body uses energy when it's at rest. In the old days, measuring your BMR was one way to determine whether you had a thyroid disease. Those who had a low BMR had an underactive thyroid. Those with a high BMR had an overactive thyroid.

Fact

Technically speaking, BMR is the rate of metabolism when you're at rest in a warm environment and have not eaten for at least twelve hours. The energy you require in this state is enough just for the vital organs such as the heart, lungs, nervous system, and kidneys. Factors that affect BMR include illness, stress, and the temperature of your environment. BMR declines with age and the loss of muscle mass.

Doctors no longer use BMR to determine your thyroid status, but a slowdown or speeding up in your metabolism is still a good indicator that something is awry with your thyroid. Getting a handle on your thyroid condition can usually put an end to this change in metabolism. But for some people, the weight problems do not go away with treatment.

A Primer on Weight

It's easy to blame your thyroid for the fact that you've recently put on some pounds. But in reality, many factors influence your body weight, and your thyroid is only one of them—albeit an important one. Other factors that influence your body weight include:

- **Genetics.** Your genes affect your appetite, your BMR, and your distribution of body fat. They may also influence your susceptibility to becoming overweight.
- **Hormones.** The body makes many hormones that regulate weight, mostly to ensure it doesn't go down. For primitive man, the problem was not enough food, so most hormones evolved to prevent weight loss.
- **Diet.** The types of food you eat and the amount you ingest have a direct effect on your weight.
- **Exercise.** The more physical activity you do, the less likely you are to gain weight.
- **Body composition.** Muscle naturally burns more calories than fat.
- **Age.** As you get older, your metabolism slows, so that you can't eat the same amount you did when you were younger without gaining weight.

People in the process of gaining weight are basically taking in more calories than they're expending. The process of becoming overweight or obese is often a slow, insidious one that you may not realize is happening until you try to squeeze into a pair of old jeans or you go shopping and realize you've jumped up a size.

Being overweight is a serious problem in the United States. Approximately two-thirds of the population is now overweight, with a third of those people being obese. This excess weight puts them at significantly higher risk for diseases such as diabetes, cancer, heart disease, and premature death.

But how do you know for sure if you really are overweight? Snug jeans or a bigger dress size are one measurement, but a more scientific method is to calculate your body mass index (BMI). BMI doesn't measure body fat, but it does tell you how your body weight relates to your height. For adults over the age of twenty, the formula is your weight in pounds divided by your height in inches squared (multiplied by itself), times 703. So if you are five foot seven and weigh 130 pounds, you have a BMI of 20.4. Here's what the number reveals:

- BMIs under 18.5 are considered underweight.
- BMIs between 18.5 and 24.9 are considered normal.
- BMIs between 25.0 and 29.9 are considered overweight.
- BMIs above 30.0 are considered obese.

Essential

For a quick calculation of your body mass index (BMI), visit the Centers for Disease Control and Prevention Web site at *www.cdc.gov/nccdphp/dnpa/bmi/calc-bmi.htm*. By simply entering your height and your weight, you'll learn your BMI in a split second.

The bottom line on weight management is simple: to lose weight, you need to expend more calories than you take in. To gain weight, you need to ingest more calories than you burn. Unfortunately, for many people, actually losing weight—and keeping it off—is an incredible challenge. The odds are stacked against most people, who must battle against hormones that prevent us from losing weight, a lifetime of ingrained habits, and lifestyles that discourage activity.

When the Thyroid Interferes

You're humming along at a healthy weight when one day you notice that your favorite pair of jeans is snug. A visit to the bathroom scale reveals what you've been dreading: you've put on weight.

To top it off, you're tired. Your skin is dry, and you're sensitive to the cold. When you finally get to the doctor, you're relieved to learn that you have hypothyroidism. Good, you think. I'll take my thyroid pill, and my weight will go back to where it was.

For some people, taking thyroid hormone replacement for hypothyroidism makes all the difference. Their excess weight disappears, their energy levels are restored to normal, and they feel well again.

But for some the solution is not so simple. Maybe you lose a few pounds initially, only to stop after a while. Or maybe the medication doesn't make a difference in your weight at all, even as other symptoms let up. In any case, having hypothyroidism can make weight loss more difficult.

Diagnostic and Treatment Challenges

For some people, it can take months, even years, before they figure out that their thyroid is at the root of their weight gain. While they're in the process of uncovering the cause of the gain, they continue to battle an increase in appetite, a craving for high-fat foods, and a lack of energy for exercise. In the meantime, their weight creeps upward.

Alert

In rare cases, hyperthyroidism can actually cause you to gain weight. If an overactive thyroid is the culprit behind your extra pounds, you are probably responding to an increase in appetite and eating too much to compensate for your body's increased energy demands.

When you are finally diagnosed, time has passed, and you've gained that much more weight. Next comes the trial-and-error period, in which you try to find the proper dosage of thyroid hormone replacement. For some, it's a matter of a few weeks before you get it right. For others, it might take several months. But again, the passage of time often means gaining more weight while you're in the process of getting properly medicated.

Too Exhausted to Move

Hypothyroidism slows you down. Your entire metabolism moves at a slower rate, so you may have little energy for even life's most mundane tasks, like preparing a meal or paying your bills. Thyroid disease can also cause joint and muscle aches that inhibit you from exercising.

When you feel this tired and achy, the idea of exercising probably seems like a monumental effort that you'd just as soon abandon in favor of the couch. The less you do, the more tired you become. So now, not only is your BMR down, but you're also getting less exercise. All this slowing down causes you to expend fewer calories than you did when your thyroid was functioning properly.

Bad Cravings

When you're tired, your body naturally craves carbohydrates and foods that give you quick energy. Unfortunately, these energy-boosting foods tend to be high in calories and fat. Many people experience these same cravings when they're depressed, bored, or going through a stressful time. Women may experience these craving when they have PMS.

But rather than truly energize you, these foods give you only a temporary boost, followed by a crash that leaves you craving more carbs. This vicious cycle—compounded by your fatigue and lack of exercise—only worsens your weight gain.

Alert

Here's one way to tame a craving—stop banning the food from your diet. According to the American Dietetic Association, an overly restrictive diet can set you up for cravings that ultimately sabotage your efforts to eat better. Instead, practice eating small portions of the tempting food, even when you're trying to lose weight.

Other Symptoms and Diseases

Having a thyroid problem slows down your digestion and can make you constipated. It can also cause swelling, which means you'll retain water. Both constipation and swelling can make you heavier.

In addition, people who have a thyroid disorder often have other endocrine abnormalities that can cause weight gain or make it hard for you to lose weight. GH deficiency as part of a pituitary problem is one problem. You may also have a condition known as insulin resistance, in which body cells have become resistant to the insulin your pancreas produces. Insulin resistance is often a precursor to diabetes and can make it hard for you to lose weight. However, people who have uncontrolled diabetes actually lose weight.

If you are being treated for thyroid disease and have attained an optimal TSH level but still can't lose weight despite all the right lifestyle choices, you may want to talk to your doctor. Your physician may need to check whether you have another condition that is inhibiting your weight loss.

Shedding the Weight

Now that you know what's behind your weight gain, you want answers to the most nagging question of all: how do I ditch these extra pounds in the face of thyroid disease?

For most people, the first thing you need to do is to get properly treated. If you have hypothyroidism, that usually means taking thyroid hormone replacement and finding the right dose. Less commonly, it might mean taking antithyroid drugs or undergoing RAI treatments to tame an overactive thyroid.

Fact

Adults aren't the only ones struggling with weight problems. Since 1980, the percentage of children six to nineteen years of age who are overweight has more than tripled, says the Centers for Disease Control and Prevention. Experts blame the problem on numerous factors, including too much TV and computer time, too many fast-food meals, and too little exercise.

The good news is, the right treatment can usually help restore you to a normal, healthy weight—or at least get you started on the right path. But losing weight often means also adopting other healthy lifestyle habits that will ensure that you not only lose the weight, but keep it off.

None of these tips are anything new. The strategies boil down to two basic habits: move more and eat less. But the types of exercise you do and the foods you choose to eat can make a big difference in how well you do in slimming down.

Move Your Body

When you're battling the fatigue and depression of hypothyroidism, exercise is probably as tempting as a vacation with pesky in-laws. To top it off, you may have other impediments to exercise. Maybe you were simply never in the habit of being active, or you find exercise boring, inconvenient, or time-consuming.

The truth is exercise is the most potent remedy you have for controlling your weight and relieving you of a thyroid-induced haze. Other perks of exercise include:

- Better sleep
- Stronger muscles
- Less tension
- Stress relief
- Less depression

On top of that, exercise enhances immunity, lowers blood pressure and cholesterol, and triggers the release of endorphins, your body's natural painkillers. Perhaps most important, exercise boosts self-confidence and helps you gain command over your health.

What Happens When You Don't Exercise?

The avoidance of exercise perpetuates a cycle that leads to greater fatigue, less activity, and more weight gain. The less you move, the weaker and smaller your muscles become. And as your muscles get smaller and weaker, your joints will become stiffer and increasingly inflexible, making it even harder for you to get the physical activity you need.

The lack of exercise can also worsen your depression, which is common in hypothyroidism. Feeling depressed, in turn, can make it harder to exercise. Next thing you know, you're trapped in a vicious cycle of fatigue, depression, and a lack of exercise, all of which can lead to unwanted weight gain.

Essential

Making exercise a regular habit can be tough for someone unaccustomed to physical activity. To make it a habit, try exercising at the same time every day. You might also want to jot down your exercise time on a calendar, enlist a partner, and set up a reward system for your efforts. Some people find it also helps to record your workouts.

That's why it's critical to always do some physical activity every day, no matter how little or how insignificant it may seem. Even short walks around the block can improve your mood, relieve your fatigue, and help you sleep better. If it's been a while since you exercised, it's best to talk to your doctor first before launching an exercise program.

Build Those Muscles

Chances are, when you think of strength training, you probably think of big, bulky men—or women—with bulging muscles. But in reality, strength training isn't only for the muscle-bound. Building muscle can benefit anyone who wants to maintain vitality, improve conditioning, and build more strength. And having more muscle mass helps ensure that you burn more calories, even at rest.

For people with hypothyroidism, strength training is important because it can help boost metabolism. The extra muscle will help keep your metabolism at a higher rate than it would if you had no muscles. And the higher your metabolism, the less likely you are to gain weight.

Certain types of strength training may be better than others for different people. The strength-training exercises you should know include:

Pilates

Although these exercises aren't new, they have recently become popular and are ideal for patients with thyroid problems. Pilates combines joint movements with muscle resistance and may involve the use of machines that look torturous but are actually energizing. The movements focus on developing and strengthening your core, which consists of your back and abdomen. Pilates also sometimes uses weights and elastic bands. Some Pilates instructors will provide individual training that can be tailored to a patient with physical impairments.

Yoga

Yoga is an ancient exercise that began in India 5,000 years ago. The movements are designed to improve flexibility, strengthen muscles, relax nerves, and promote circulation. Some stretches and poses can be quite rigorous. Yoga can be done in a group or individually.

Water Resistance Training

Using water as resistance is another way to build strength, and a good one for people with muscle and joint pain. The water provides natural support for the joints, making a water workout less likely to cause injury and pain.

Cardiovascular Exercise

Whether it's a brisk walk, a long bike ride, or a kickboxing class, anything that gets the heart pumping can strengthen your heart and increase your endurance. When you engage in cardiovascular exercise, you breathe harder, so your lungs are working harder, too. These exercises also improve blood flow; aid in weight loss; and lower blood pressure, triglycerides, and LDL cholesterol, the bad cholesterol. In addition, cardio workouts can minimize depression, reduce stress, and improve sleep—all of which help stave off weight gain and perpetuate weight loss.

Question

Won't exercise make me hungrier and cause me to eat more?
It's true, high-intensity exercise definitely does stimulate the appetite, according to a study in the American Journal of Clinical Nutrition. But moderate exercise—the kind you're more likely to do when you have hypothyroidism—does not produce the same effects.

For someone who has hypothyroidism, getting a cardiovascular workout might seem too daunting, especially if you're new to exercise. The thought of even driving to a pool might seem too exhausting, much less getting in and swimming laps. That's why it's important to choose your cardio workout carefully. When you're in the throes of serious fatigue, it'll be hard to muster the energy for a rigorous aerobic workout. Instead, look for low-impact activities that you really enjoy. The pleasure of an activity will help ensure that you'll do it again, day after day.

A Word on Walking

One of the best cardio exercises you can do is walking. It's safe, convenient, and easy, and requires no special equipment. It doesn't involve a pricey gym membership, and you can do it virtually anywhere. You don't even need any special training. All you do need is a good pair of walking shoes. Walking is also unlikely to cause injuries that might deter you from exercising in the future.

If you decide that walking is the best exercise for you, then by all means, give it a try. Always wear a good pair of well-fitting shoes that provide adequate support. Replace old shoes that are unevenly worn, which can cause an imbalance in your footing and lead to muscle pain.

When you do start walking, go slowly and resist the urge to walk lengthy distances. If you feel stiff, do some gentle stretches before heading out. Don't push yourself too hard, which can lead to injuries that interfere with workouts. Exercising regularly is more important than getting a single strenuous workout.

Essential

The perks of exercise aren't always immediately obvious. One way to track your progress and see the benefits is to keep an exercise diary. Record the date and time, the activity you do, the duration of your workout, and how you feel after you exercise and the rest of the day.

While you walk, make sure to breathe as normally as possible. To stay safe, walk in well-populated areas or carry a cell phone, in case of emergency. If it's hot, carry a water bottle so you can stay hydrated. Finish the walk with a cool-down walk and some gentle stretching.

Choose Your Foods Wisely

Exercise and healthy eating go hand in hand when it comes to weight loss. You simply can't lose weight if you exercise but then spend the evening noshing on potato chips in front of the TV. Likewise, it's hard to keep the weight off just by eating less, doing no exercise. So when it comes to eating for weight loss, the key is making the right choices and keeping portion sizes to a minimum.

Healthy Food Choices

When you're trying to lose weight, the foods you choose to eat play a big role in how successful your efforts are. A diet rich in saturated fats, cholesterol, and added sugars will do little to help you shed the extra pounds. Instead, you need to eat foods that help you feel full and provide your body with the maximum amount of nutrients.

Truth is, there is no one diet just for patients with thyroid disorders. There is also no food that works to magically lower your weight. Instead, your diet should be composed of foods from all the important food groups—proteins, complex carbohydrates, low-fat dairy, and fruits and vegetables. At the same time, a healthy diet also makes room for occasional indulgences like dessert or a candy bar. Here are some general guidelines to help you eat wisely for weight loss:

- Choose complex carbohydrates over simple carbohydrates. Complex carbs such as whole wheat pasta, vegetables, and fruits are high in fiber, which will fill you up for longer.
- Select fats carefully. Beware of foods high in saturated fats. These foods include processed meats, high-fat cuts of meat, and whole-milk dairy foods. Instead, make the switch to low-fat versions. Also avoid polyunsaturated fats, found in cakes and cookies. Monounsaturated fats, found in olive oil and avocados, are your healthiest options.

- Eat healthy proteins. Consider alternatives to red meat, such as skinless chicken, fish, turkey, beans, nuts, seeds, and tofu.
- Watch your alcohol intake. Alcoholic drinks are high in calories and low in nutritional value.
- Drink plenty of water, preferably eight glasses a day. Proper hydration keeps your body functioning at its best.

Portion Control

In a society that puts a premium on getting a good deal, it's tempting to put monetary concerns ahead of your health. After all, everyone wants to get the biggest bang for his buck. But in reality, ordering jumbo-size fast-food meals and indulging at the all-you-can-eat buffet quickly sabotages any weight-loss efforts.

 Alert

People desperate to lose weight are vulnerable to scams touting quick weight-loss programs. In reality, weight loss takes time and patience, especially if you want the weight loss to stick. So resist the urge to buy into empty promises. If something sounds too good to be true, it probably is.

If you truly want to lose weight, give a lot of thought to portion control. Plan out strategies that will help prevent you from overeating. Some good ideas from the American Dietetic Association include:

- Eat off a smaller plate.
- Nibble on some low-cal foods before the actual meal. Raw veggies or a small salad will help quell your appetite.
- When dining out, put away half the meal before you even begin.
- Get in the habit of splitting desserts, if you do indulge.
- Set down the fork as soon as you feel full.

Create Healthy Eating Habits

Many people overeat out of habit. Perhaps you're accustomed to taking seconds every night at the dinner table. Or maybe you've always snacked in front of the TV. For some people, breaking these bad habits can make an enormous difference in weight loss. Among the bad habits:

Emotional Overeating

Many people eat when they're bored, stressed, upset, or sad. If your eating habits are driven by emotion, you need to find substitute activities for tough emotional times. Instead of eating, try taking a walk, calling a friend, or tending your garden.

Meal Skipping

In an effort to cut back on calories—or simply because they're running late—some people skip meals, especially breakfast. But meal skipping, especially breakfast, is a no-no for weight loss. Studies have shown that people who don't eat breakfast are more likely to gain weight. Eating on a regular schedule will help prevent a ravenous appetite later on that leads to overeating.

Mindless Eating

Some people eat because the bowl of M&Ms is sitting there or because their child left a few French fries on her plate. If you're trying to lose weight, these mindless moments can quickly add up to caloric overload. Instead, eat only when you're hungry.

Eating Too Fast

Stuffing the food into your mouth without really tasting it can also sabotage weight-loss efforts. It usually takes twenty minutes to feel full, but by then you've already eaten too much. Try eating slowly, which can help you feel full before you take a second helping. For more tips on mindful eating, see Chapter 20. Mindful eating should be part of everyone's lifestyle, not just those trying to lose weight.

When You Can't Gain Weight

In people who have hyperthyroidism, inexplicable weight loss is a common problem. As the amount of thyroid hormone increases, the activity of your body cells speeds up, causing you to burn more energy than normal even without additional physical activity.

In some people, this extra energy burn causes a parallel increase in appetite. But for others, the appetite boost actually causes weight gain when the calories you ingest surpass your level of physical activity.

Everyone tells you you're lucky to be so thin, but in reality, being too thin poses its own set of health problems. You may be vulnerable to serious injuries if you fall, and you are also at higher risk for infection. In addition, being underweight can cause fatigue, irritability, and the inability to concentrate. Here are some tips from the ADA:

- Try five or six small meals instead of three bigger ones.
- Avoid drinking too much during meals, which can fill you up.
- Exercise regularly, which will stimulate your appetite and boost your body's energy demands.
- Enhance the appeal of your foods with more color, texture, and aroma.
- Make mealtime pleasurable by dining with friends.
- Take a walk before eating to stimulate appetite.

And whatever you do, make sure to continue loading up on healthy foods. Being underweight is not an opportunity to indulge in excess amounts of high-fat foods. Thin people will face the same health risks as heavy people if they eat too much saturated fats, cholesterol, and sugars.

CHAPTER 16

Thyroid Disease and Children

Unlike some diseases that tend to occur with age, thyroid disorders do not discriminate against the young. Thyroid disorders can strike children, even newborns, just as easily as they can occur in adulthood. While thyroid disease in children used to be a common cause of mental retardation, today there is greater awareness—and earlier screenings—to detect thyroid disease before it poses a serious problem. Still, thyroid problems can occur.

Challenges in Children

By now, you're well aware of what it takes to diagnose, treat, and manage thyroid disease. In a child who develops thyroid disease, however, new challenges emerge. For starters, children are usually less aware of their symptoms. Infants obviously can't describe the symptoms they're experiencing, but even an older child with thyroid disease may not be aware that something is wrong. That means vigilant adults—parents and doctors—need to be on the lookout for signs of thyroid disease.

Detecting thyroid disease in children is critical to their health and well-being, both now and in the future. They're still in the process of growing and require just the right amount of thyroid hormone for the normal development of vital organs, including the brain and heart. A consequence of untreated hypothyroidism in infants, for example, can be mental retardation. Hyperthyroidism in older children can cause serious behavioral issues that affect their academic performance. A long delay in the treatment of hypothyroidism can lead to stunted growth and a delay in puberty.

Managing thyroid disease is also considerably more difficult in children. Unlike adults, who can grasp the consequences of not taking their medication, some children may balk at the idea of taking a daily pill. Others may have difficulty swallowing a pill. Yet, taking medication consistently is essential to the successful management of thyroid disease.

Although many of the thyroid problems that occur in children are the same as those that occur in adults, it's important to revisit these conditions in this chapter. Not all the treatments that work well for adults are advisable for children. It's also important to understand the impact of thyroid disease on a child's growth and development, especially in families where autoimmune diseases of the thyroid and other thyroid disorders are common.

Congenital Hypothyroidism

Every year in the United States, approximately 1 in 4,000 babies is born with congenital hypothyroidism. The term congenital simply means that the condition is present at birth. A baby who is born with hypothyroidism is at serious risk for mental retardation and growth problems. The good news is that since the 1970s, most industrialized countries, including the United States and Canada, have screened newborns for thyroid disease with a simple blood test that has helped to significantly reduce the risk for retardation in babies born with hypothyroidism.

For this test, a drop of blood is drawn from your baby's heel about twenty-four to seventy-two hours after birth. The blood is placed on a special filter paper that can measure your baby's TSH levels. If TSH is high, your physician will immediately start treating your baby with levothyroxine to replace the missing thyroid hormone that her body isn't naturally producing. If TSH is slightly elevated, your doctor may test your baby's free T4 levels first before starting treatment.

Some doctors may also do an X-ray of your baby's legs to look at the ends of the bones, which may appear immature in babies with congenital hypothyroidism. Doctors may also do a thyroid scan to determine the location or absence of the thyroid gland (see below).

Fact

According to the March of Dimes, congenital hypothyroidism is the most common disorder identified by screening in newborns. Other diseases include phenylketonuria (PKU), in which the baby can't process a part of an amino acid called phenylalanine, and galactosemia, in which the baby can't convert a sugar called galactose into glucose. All three conditions can cause mental retardation. Incidentally, the same blood sample can screen for at least fifty-five different diseases.

Sometimes, follow-up blood tests will show that your baby's thyroid has resumed normal function. But because of the seriousness of untreated hypothyroidism, some doctors will opt to go ahead and continue treatment until future tests show that the child is euthyroid.

In rare cases, your baby's inadequate thyroid hormone may be a temporary problem called transient congenital hypothyroidism. This condition may occur if the mother was exposed to excess iodine during pregnancy, or if she took too much antithyroid medication for hyperthyroidism. In both instances, the baby's thyroid is temporarily blocked from producing enough thyroid hormone. An iodine deficiency can also cause transient congenital hypothyroidism. Even more rare, transient congenital hypothyroidism may be the result of excess amounts of TSI found in Graves' disease in the mother.

Alert

> To give your baby levothyroxine, crush the tablet and dissolve it in water, then feed it with a dropper. Do not mix levothyroxine in soy-based infant formula; this can inhibit absorption of the drug.

If the hypothyroidism is transient, your baby's thyroid gland will correct itself over time, and thyroid hormone levels will eventually become normal. Transient congenital hypothyroidism is generally more common in premature or low-birth-weight babies. But it's impossible to know whether your child has transient or permanent hypothyroidism, which is why all babies who have low levels of TSH are treated with thyroid hormone replacement.

Causes

The most common cause of congenital hypothyroidism is an ectopic thyroid. Just like an ectopic pregnancy—in which the fertilized egg starts to grow outside the uterus—an ectopic thyroid grows in an inappropriate location. Because the ectopic thyroid is not properly located, these glands generally don't function correctly and fail to produce enough thyroid hormone.

Development of the thyroid gland begins in the first trimester of pregnancy, when the first remnants of thyroid tissue in the back of the tongue start making the gradual descent to the base of the neck. There, a healthy gland grows and forms, then starts churning out thyroid hormone that aids in the development of the fetus. But if that tissue doesn't migrate properly, the thyroid gland is said to be ectopic.

In most cases of ectopic thyroid, the thyroid gland develops where it originates, in the back of the tongue. This type of development is called a lingual thyroid. On occasion, these misplaced thyroid glands actually do produce enough thyroid hormone, and the patient may not even know that anything is wrong.

Lingual thyroid is more common in girls than boys. Though most are small and less than a centimeter, some can grow to four centimeters. In some patients, a lingual thyroid can interfere with swallowing or breathing.

The majority of babies born with a lingual thyroid go on to develop hypothyroidism. Treatment to prevent hypothyroidism usually involves suppressing TSH levels so that the lingual thyroid does not grow. If it gets too big or affects swallowing, your child may require surgery. People with lingual thyroid usually undergo regular monitoring of thyroid hormone levels.

Essential

Lingual thyroid isn't detected only in children. In rare cases, they may not become apparent until adulthood, even into your seventies. Signs and symptoms are generally the same—shortness of breath and difficulty swallowing.

Some babies with congenital hypothyroidism are born without a thyroid gland or one that is smaller than normal. In some cases, a baby has hypothyroidism because the mother had a deficiency of iodine, a situation that is rare in the United States. Some babies may lack an enzyme required for iodine metabolism, which causes a deficit in thyroid hormone production. Babies born without this enzyme may also be deaf.

Signs and Symptoms

Most babies born with hypothyroidism look perfectly normal at birth. That's why the screening process is essential for detecting babies who lack adequate thyroid hormone. But some babies may actually have one or more symptoms, including:

- Decreased birth weight
- Puffy face

- Swollen tongue
- A hoarse cry
- Cold hands and feet
- Persistent constipation and a bloated abdomen
- Prolonged jaundice
- Lack of energy and constant fatigue
- Poor muscle tone
- Little or no growth over time

Although the newborn screening has become routine, parents should still be on the lookout for suspicious symptoms. And if you come from a family where thyroid disease is prevalent, it doesn't hurt to ask about the screening to make sure it's done.

Cretinism

Children without enough thyroid hormone are at serious risk for cretinism, a condition that causes severe retardation in both physical and mental development. Cretinism is common in regions of the world where iodine is deficient, goiter is endemic, and screening is not performed. Worldwide, cretinism is the most common cause of mental retardation.

Fact

According to MedicineNet.com, the word cretin may have come from the Old French term chretien, meaning "Christian." Fleeing persecution, Christians moved into the Pyrenees valleys, where a lack of iodine caused them to have children with congenital hypothyroidism. Another theory is that the word could have come from cretura, meaning "creature," or creta, meaning "chalk" or "pale."

People who have cretinism suffer numerous problems. Growth is permanently stunted, and an adult will be well below normal height.

Cretinism also causes the skin to be thick and flabby, and waxy in color. Most children with cretinism have a flattened nose and a protruding stomach. Gait and speech are notably slow, and intellectual development is seriously limited.

Thyroglossal Duct Cysts

You're bathing your toddler one day when you notice a strange lump at the base of your baby's throat that you've never seen before. Some children are born with a thyroglossal duct cyst, a developmental abnormality that occurs during the formation of the thyroid gland in the first trimester of pregnancy.

When the thyroid tissue descends from the base of the tongue toward the base of the throat, it passes through a duct. Normally, this duct disintegrates on its own and disappears. But in some children, remnants of the duct remain, causing cysts that appear as a lump in the front of the neck. The duct is rarely apparent in babies, whose excess fat conceals the duct. But once the child is older and slims down, a duct cyst becomes more obvious. In some cases, a thyroglossal duct cyst isn't discovered until much later.

If you discover a lump in the throat of your toddler, it's critical to have it evaluated by a doctor. A thyroglossal duct cyst needs to be distinguished from a nodule. To do that, your doctor may ask your child to swallow some water and to stick out his tongue. Both actions will cause the cyst to move upward since it is still connected to the tongue. Your doctor may do blood tests and a thyroid scan to measure thyroid function. He may also do an ultrasound to examine the duct cyst.

Treatment usually involves surgery. If the thyroglossal duct cyst is infected, your child will need antibiotics first to eliminate the infection. The cyst may also need to be drained.

The most common procedure is called the Sistrunk operation, which has been shown to decrease the recurrence of cysts. An incision is made in the center of the neck near the lump in a natural crease, and the entire cyst is removed as well as the cyst tract and a small part of the hyoid bone, which supports the tongue. The procedure is done under general anesthesia. The surgical site is then sutured to minimize visible scarring.

L. Essential

The biggest problem with a thyroglossal duct cyst is the risk for infection. Bacteria from the mouth (which is prevalent) can invade the cyst, causing redness and tenderness. An infected cyst should not be operated on.

After removal, the cyst will be closely examined for thyroid tissue, which can raise the risk for cancer. It's extremely rare, however, to have cancer of the cyst.

Acquired Hypothyroidism

In some children, hypothyroidism does not become apparent until much later on. This condition may appear in early childhood, but is usually more common in young teens. Just like in adults, hypothyroidism in children can cause fatigue, weight gain, constipation, and dryness. It can also affect your child's performance in school, making it hard for her to concentrate and do well.

But in kids, the ramifications of hypothyroidism are more serious since inadequate thyroid hormone can stunt growth and development. In some children, hypothyroidism can delay puberty, though in some cases, it can actually cause premature puberty.

The vast majority of children who develop hypothyroidism have Hashimoto's disease, an autoimmune condition we discuss in detail in Chapter 6. But in some cases, the hypothyroidism may be the result of previously undetected defects in the manufacture of thyroid hormone, or of tumors on the pituitary gland or hypothalamus, which can affect the production of TSH.

Hypothyroidism may also be the result of radiation treatments. Children who receive radiation aimed at regions near the thyroid gland or at parts of the brain involved in thyroid hormone production are vulnerable to developing hypothyroidism.

Like adult hypothyroidism and congenital hypothyroidism, treatment is fairly simple and involves replacing the missing thyroid hormone. Dosage depends primarily on the child's age and body weight.

Essential

Some children are at greater risk for developing Hashimoto's and should be checked in regular intervals. Children with type 1 diabetes, Down's syndrome, or a family history of thyroid disease are all at greater risk for Hashimoto's. Girls with Turner syndrome, a chromosomal disease, are also at greater risk.

Hyperthyroidism

Children are naturally active, but when excess activity is accompanied by a rapid heart rate, trouble breathing, and chronic nervousness, your child may have hyperthyroidism. As in adults, hyperthyroidism is much less common in children than hypothyroidism is. Estimates show that it occurs in 1 of every 5,000 children.

When hyperthyroidism occurs in newborns, it is often a temporary problem caused by a mother having Graves' disease. When a mother has Graves' disease, TSIs are transferred across the placenta to the fetus, causing the baby to produce larger than normal amounts of thyroid hormone. Symptoms of hyperthyroidism include a rapid heart rate, an enlarged thyroid gland, poor weight gain, bulging eyes, and irritability. Until the condition goes away, which may take a few months, your baby may be given an antithyroid drug to control her symptoms. She may also be given a beta-blocker to slow down her heart rate.

Hyperthyroidism in older children resembles that which occurs in adults—nervousness, anxiety, irritability, trouble breathing, and a rapid heart rate are all common symptoms. Some kids may have behavior problems at school and suffer in their academic performance.

Alert

Treatment for a baby with hyperthyroidism is critical. Left untreated, hyperthyroidism in a baby can be fatal. A woman who has Graves' disease must be closely monitored throughout her pregnancy. Babies born to moms with Graves' must be routinely checked after birth.

But in children, hyperthyroidism may also cause accelerated growth. The effects of this faster growth are usually subtle. For example, over the course of a year or two, the hyperthyroid child's height may climb from the fiftieth percentile to the seventy-fifth. Your child may also have trouble gaining weight and drop to a lower percentile in body weight in spite of a marked increase in appetite. Hyperthyroidism can also delay puberty, or cause it to slow. In girls who have already started their periods, hyperthyroidism can cause their periods to slow or stop completely.

Like in adults, the most common cause of hyperthyroidism in children is Graves' disease, which is discussed in detail in Chapter 9. During pregnancy, maternal antibodies cross the placenta and stimulate the baby's developing thyroid gland, causing it to produce more thyroid hormone.

Treating Graves' disease in children is slightly more complex than it is in adults. Although children have the same treatment options that adults do, some doctors worry that treatment with RAI could raise the risk of thyroid cancer, as well as infertility, later on. For that reason, initial treatment for a child usually involves antithyroid drugs. In many cases, after a few years of treatment, the disease usually goes into remission.

But if the disease is severe and cannot be resolved with drugs, your child may require a more definitive treatment such as surgery or RAI treatments. Concerns about the safety of RAI are based on reports linking external radiation to thyroid cancer. But as of now, there is no hard evidence showing that the low doses involved in RAI actually cause cancer or infertility.

If a child does undergo RAI or surgery, there is a good chance she will become hypothyroid and will require thyroid hormone replacement for the rest of her life.

Thyroiditis

Your child is complaining of a sore throat and suffering from a low-grade fever. A throat culture rules out strep throat, but the pain persists. A check of her throat reveals that her thyroid gland is slightly swollen. A blood test may show that your child is suffering from subacute thyroiditis.

Essential

If your child has chronic thyroiditis that lasts more than a few weeks, she may have an autoimmune disorder, meaning that her thyroid gland contains lymphocytes. Symptoms of chronic thyroiditis vary. The child may have a diffuse goiter, and may be either hypothyroid or hyperthyroid. Some children become permanently hypothyroid. Others may go into remission and become euthyroid.

After a brief viral illness, your child may develop subacute thyroiditis, which causes neck pain, goiter, and sometimes fever, hoarseness, and trouble swallowing. Children can also develop silent thyroiditis, a condition characterized only by symptoms of hyperthyroidism and inflammation of the thyroid. In addition, children may get acute suppurative thyroiditis, in which bacteria invade the thyroid gland

and trigger inflammation. With acute suppurative thyroiditis, the child may feel a lot of pain, a fever, and chills.

Treatment for thyroiditis depends on the type you have. Subacute and silent thyroiditis usually involve bed rest and nonsteroidal anti-inflammatories to relieve the pain. Acute suppurative thyroiditis requires antibiotics to wipe out the bacteria. Most cases of thyroiditis will resolve on their own after a few weeks.

Goiters and Nodules

Although goiters and nodules are more common in older adults, they can occur in children as well. Both are more common in girls than boys. And children get goiters and nodules for most of the same reasons that adults do, although multinodular goiter is rare in children. Kids are more likely to have diffuse goiters caused by autoimmune disease.

Goiters

Like adults, children living in regions of the world deficient in iodine are prone to developing goiters. Inadequate iodine stimulates the release of TSH, which, in turn, causes the thyroid gland to become enlarged as it struggles to produce more thyroid hormone. Here in the United States, the most common cause for a goiter in children is Hashimoto's disease. In fact, a goiter may be the first and most obvious sign of the disorder that parents will notice. The neck may appear full or swollen, and the child may say she feels pressure in her neck or throat.

Children may also develop goiters as the result of thyroiditis, inflammation of the thyroid gland, or Graves' disease, which causes hyperthyroidism. In some cases, a child may develop a goiter but still have normal thyroid function, which is a euthyroid goiter.

Treatment for goiters in children involves treating the underlying disease. For instance, thyroid hormone replacement given for Hashimoto's usually causes the goiter to shrink. But if a goiter is euthyroid, small, and not causing any problems with breathing or swallowing, your doctor may do nothing and simply keep an eye on it.

Nodules

Thyroid nodules are less common in children than in adults, but when they do occur, they're slightly more likely to be malignant than nodules in adults are. Close examination and testing of the nodule is critical to determine the cause of the nodule. Fortunately, the majority of nodules in kids will turn out to be benign.

Although rare, some older children may develop a toxic adenoma, nodules that produce their own supply of thyroid hormone as a result of faulty TSH receptor. When the amount of thyroid hormone becomes significantly elevated, your child will eventually experience symptoms of hyperthyroidism. An RAIU test and scan will reveal that the nodule is hot and absorbing iodine.

Essential

To the untrained eye (or hand), it's easy to mistake a swollen lymph node for a thyroid nodule. After all, both are on the neck. Swollen lymph nodes tend to occur when there is an infection and are located more on the sides of the neck. A thyroid nodule would be farther down, near the base of the neck. Always check with your doctor if you feel any lump.

In general, a small toxic adenoma is best treated with radioactive iodine, while a larger one may require surgery. Antithyroid drugs will have little effect since toxic adenomas do not go into remission.

Thyroid Cancer in Kids

Thyroid cancer is very rare in children, but when it does occur, it can be more aggressive than it is in adults, often spreading into nearby tissue such as the lymph nodes. The most common type of thyroid cancer in children is papillary cancer.

Because the cancer can be more aggressive in kids, treatment must be equally aggressive. Surgery to remove the entire gland is followed up with RAI ablation to destroy any cancerous cells that have migrated elsewhere in the body. Afterward, the child is given thyroid hormone replacement, a medication that he will need to take for the rest of his life. And like adults, children who have had thyroid cancer need lifelong monitoring. Routine blood tests, thyroglobulin tests, and whole body scans are done regularly to ensure that the cancer has not returned. Getting your child in the habit of following up on these tests will help instill a lifetime of vigilance. For more information on cancer, refer back to Chapter 11.

Early Testing for Medullary Cancer

Medullary cancer is a specific form of thyroid cancer that is passed on through your genes. Approximately 20 percent of all people who have it carry an abnormal gene they inherited from a parent, but almost all children who have medullary cancer have this abnormal gene. Babies born to a parent who has this gene can be tested at birth with a screening test.

Fact

Children who inherit mutations of the gene are best off getting their thyroid glands surgically removed before age eight, according to a study published in the *New England Journal of Medicine* in 2005. The study found that five years after the procedure, the kids who had surgery before age eight had no evidence of thyroid cancer, while those who were older than eight at surgery did show signs of cancer.

Unlike most other cancers, having the gene for thyroid cancer does mean your child is destined to get thyroid cancer. That's why surgery is necessary. Having surgery while your child is young ensures that your child won't get medullary thyroid cancer.

Meeting the Challenges

We started this chapter with a discussion of the unique challenges facing children who experience thyroid disease. Although thyroid disease can be more complex and difficult in kids, parents who are vigilant can steer their children toward proper diagnosis and treatment and a lifetime of routine monitoring and adherence to medications. The key—as with any parental task—is to be consistent and persistent. Here are some ways to help your child cope with thyroid disease:

Instill Compliance

Let's face it: No one really likes to take medication. It's one more thing to remember, and children simply don't want to be bothered. But if your child has hypothyroidism—or any other condition for that matter—that requires taking a pill regularly, compliance is essential to her health. Not taking your daily pill is simply not an option. Here are some ways to make sure your child takes her pill:

- Discuss the importance of taking the medication in age-appropriate ways that your child will understand.
- Place the pill in a colorful container with the days of the week marked.
- Ask your child to mark an x on the calendar each day she takes her pill.
- If your child has trouble swallowing pills, consider crushing her pill and incorporating it into food. But some pills cannot be crushed and must be taken whole. Check with your doctor or pharmacist first.
- Get in the habit of taking the pill at the same time every day and in the same way. The repetition will reinforce the habit.

Honesty Is the Best Policy

Breaking the news to your child that she is sick is painful for any parent, especially if the illness is life-threatening. But trying to shield her from the truth about her medical condition won't help. Without knowing the truth, your child may resort to her imagination, which will only stoke her fears. And chances are, your child already knows that something is going on if she's going to the doctor more frequently and can see the anxious expressions on her parents' faces.

What you say, how you say it, and when you choose to divulge your child's illness is up to you. You know your child best. But whatever you do or say should be age appropriate. For instance, a five-year-old is not apt to understand that thyroid cancer is potentially deadly, so you may not need to even discuss that aspect of the disease. But a teenager is usually well aware that cancer can be fatal, so you may need to discuss the survival rates associated with thyroid cancer.

Be Vigilant

Chances are, if you're reading this book, you either have thyroid disease or have a family member who does. Knowing that thyroid problems are in your family should make you more vigilant about these disorders in your children. As we noted early on, children aren't always aware that they're anxious, nervous, or sluggish. They don't always notice that they've become sensitive to cold or heat or that their skin is unusually dry or moist. And the impact of thyroid disease on your child's growth isn't always immediately apparent (which is why you should keep track of your child's height and weight).

That's why it's important to be vigilant and to pay attention to your child's health. Don't be afraid to prod your child for more details about how she is feeling, especially if she doesn't seem to be acting right. Report anything suspicious to your pediatrician. And be sure to tell your child's doctor if you do have a family history of thyroid disease. Simple details and information can go a long way toward a quick and accurate diagnosis.

CHAPTER 17

Thyroid Disease and Aging

The risk of almost any illness rises with age, and thyroid disease is no exception. But detecting thyroid disease also becomes more difficult in older people since symptoms are easily confused with physical changes that occur with advancing age. In this chapter, you'll take a look at how thyroid problems appear in the elderly, treatment concerns that arise with age, and how thyroid disease affects mental health in older patients.

The Thyroid and the Elderly

For many older adults, it's not unusual to experience some mild forgetfulness, fatigue, and difficulty sleeping. You may also feel somewhat depressed and find that you've become intolerant of the cold. Your skin and hair may be dry, and you may not have the appetite you once did. You may also notice that you have heart palpitations and some pains in your chest, especially when lugging groceries or climbing stairs.

None of these symptoms sound unusual to someone who is getting older. And if you're like many older adults, you simply chalk up these myriad ailments to advancing age. But in reality, these signs and symptoms could also be clues that you have thyroid disease.

Statistics show that thyroid disease—particularly hypothyroidism—is more common in older adults than it is in younger people. While younger women are more likely to have problems with their immune system, putting them at risk for Hashimoto's or Graves' disease, men start catching up with women as they get older. The ability of the thyroid gland to produce enough thyroid hormone also can diminish with age. Consider these statistics from the AACE:

- One out of every five women over the age of sixty-five has a higher than normal TSH level, an indication of hypothyroidism.
- Approximately 15 percent of all patients diagnosed with hyperthyroidism are over the age of sixty.
- By age sixty, 17 percent of women and 9 percent of men have hypothyroidism. In numbers, that's about 5.7 million women and 2.7 million men.
- Approximately 20 to 25 percent of Americans over the age of sixty suffer from symptoms of mental illness, such as depression, which might actually be attributed to thyroid disease.

Often, it takes a vigilant doctor to catch thyroid disease in an elderly patient. Most physicians—and patients, too—are more apt to suspect heart disease, depression, and aging as the cause of symptoms. But if you have a personal or family history of thyroid or autoimmune disease, you may want to consider your thyroid as a possible culprit.

Hypothyroidism

It's not at all uncommon for an older adult to develop hypothyroidism. It's also not uncommon for the condition to be undiagnosed or incorrectly diagnosed. In fact, according to the ATA, one in four patients in nursing homes may have undiagnosed hypothyroidism.

Symptoms of hypothyroidism in older adults are the same as they are for younger people—weight gain, dry skin, intolerance for the cold, depression, and fatigue, for instance. But older patients are less likely to have multiple symptoms. Many of the classic symptoms are often absent, and in some cases, they may have only one symptom, such as memory loss, which is easily dismissed as a sign of old age.

So when does a physician begin to consider the possibility of thyroid disease? That depends largely on the physician, his training, experience, and knowledge. Sometimes, an in-depth conversation with the patient will reveal a family history of thyroid disease. Or perhaps the patient will reveal a long-ago treatment for a bout of hyperthyroidism. Perhaps the conversation will uncover a distant memory of surgery or radiation performed on the neck. Once a physician suspects the thyroid, he will order a test to see whether there is an elevated TSH level.

Essential

Postmenopausal women who are taking hormone replacement therapy (HRT) may require higher doses of levothyroxine than women not taking HRT. The synthetic estrogen in HRT causes an increase in the production of thyroid binding globulin, which can cause a reduction in thyroid hormone in the bloodstream.

If your TSH levels are indeed high, and you're experiencing symptoms of hypothyroidism, your doctor will probably start treating you with thyroid hormone replacement. Older patients, especially those with heart disease, generally start on a lower dose so that the medication does not stress the heart. The lower dosage will give your body the time it needs to adjust to the medication. For more information on hypothyroidism, see Chapter 4.

Hyperthyroidism

Hyperthyroidism is rare in older adults, but when it does occur, it's often the result of a toxic multinodular goiter. In some cases, the cause is Graves' disease, while in others, it may be the result of taking too much thyroid hormone replacement for the treatment of hypothyroidism.

As with hypothyroidism, the signs and symptoms of hyperthyroidism are easily confused with those of aging or conditions associated with age. To make matters more challenging, hyperthyroidism in older adults sometimes produces none of the telltale signs that you see in younger adults. For example, while younger adults may experience tremors, nervousness, and intolerance for heat, these symptoms are sometimes nonexistent in older adults.

Alert

Unintentional weight loss in an older adult can lead to serious consequences such as muscle wasting, weakened immunity, depression, and higher rates of infection. Weight loss in the elderly is also associated with a higher risk of death.

Older people who do have symptoms of hyperthyroidism will often experience weight loss. They may also be more irritable and tired. One study found that older adults with hyperthyroidism are more prone to atrial fibrillations and anorexia than younger people. But again, all these symptoms are common in older adults and may be easily dismissed as signs of old age.

Sometimes, older people with hyperthyroidism may develop a condition known as apathetic hyperthyroidism. Approximately 10 to 15 percent of all older adults with hyperthyroidism have this form of the disease. Rather than becoming nervous, jittery, and restless, people with apathetic hyperthyroidism are lethargic, weak, and depressed. Because these symptoms resemble a psychiatric problem, the patient may be misdiagnosed at first, possibly with depression.

Once the disease is detected, older people with hyperthyroidism have the same treatment options as younger adults, namely antithyroid medications and RAI treatment. Surgery is less likely to be considered because of its inherent risks to older people, who are generally more frail. Those who are given RAI can be first treated with antithyroid drugs to bring thyroid hormone levels under better control. They may also be given beta-blockers to tame any bothersome symptoms.

Subclinical Thyroid Disease

Like anyone, older adults can sometimes develop a mild or subclinical case of hypo- or hyperthyroidism. With subclinical hypothyroidism, your TSH levels may be only slightly elevated, but you may be experiencing mild symptoms of hypothyroidism. Subclinical hypothyroidism is actually more common in older people than it is in younger adults.

With subclinical hyperthyroidism, your TSH levels may be normal or just slightly reduced. You may also have symptoms of hyperthyroidism.

The impact of subclinical hypo- and hyperthyroidism is unclear. Some studies have suggested that subclinical hypothyroidism can raise your risk for atherosclerosis and heart disease independently of cholesterol. One study in the *Archives of Internal Medicine* in 2005 found that the incidence of heart failure was significantly higher in people aged seventy to seventy-nine with elevated TSH levels than it was in those who were euthyroid.

Essential

The management of subclinical thyroid disease may depend on whether you have pre-existing heart disease or another serious heart condition. If you do, you may need to undergo more frequent testing once an abnormal TSH is detected.

The question, however, is whether to treat an older person with subclinical thyroid disease. Not all patients necessarily need or benefit from treatment of subclinical disease. Some patients may recover on their own without any medical intervention. Sometimes, treatment is even potentially harmful. Too much thyroid hormone in the treatment of hypothyroidism, for instance, can cause bone loss, a worsening of heart disease, or the onset of heart problems.

Without any clear-cut guidelines, doctors have been left to decide each case individually. Some doctors may decide to treat patients who have symptoms. Others may treat patients who show persistently abnormal TSH tests. Still others may treat only those who test positive for autoantibodies showing the presence of an autoimmune disease. In any case, if you have subclinical hypo- or hyperthyroidism, it will be up to your doctor to decide how you will be treated.

Risks of Thyroid Disease in Elderly

It isn't easy to detect thyroid disease in the elderly. But left untreated, thyroid disease can have serious ramifications for older adults, especially women in their postmenopausal years. Inadequate or excess amounts of thyroid hormone can speed the rate of bone loss, promote the buildup of cholesterol, and raise your risk of heart disease.

Osteoporosis

Bones naturally weaken with age, especially in women who lose the protective effects of estrogen after menopause. But some people develop a condition called osteoporosis, which is low bone density. Osteoporosis is a silent disease that produces no symptoms, and most people won't know they have it unless they suffer a fracture. Approximately 10 million people in the United States have osteoporosis, 8 million of them women. Each year, approximately 1.5 million American adults suffer an osteoporosis-related fracture.

Throughout life, our bones are in the constant process of breaking down and rebuilding. This process is achieved through the activity of osteoclasts, which break down the bone, and osteoblasts, which restore the bone. Having too much thyroid hormone accelerates the breakdown of bone by stimulating the osteoclasts. As a result, the osteoclasts go into overdrive without any activity from the osteoblasts, which are not affected by the excess thyroid hormone and so will not compensate for the bone loss.

⌶. Essential

> Women over age sixty-five should get 1,500 mg of calcium a day. If you're postmenopausal, regardless of whether you are taking HRT, you should also aim for 1,500 mg. Women between the ages of twenty-five and fifty should get 1,000 mg a day. Ideally, you should break up your calcium intake through the day since your body can absorb only about 600 mg at a time. Good dietary sources include low-fat milk, yogurt, and cheese.

Proper treatment of hyperthyroidism to reduce the amount of thyroid hormone in your body puts an end to this destructive process. You can also take measures to minimize bone loss by eating adequate amounts of calcium and vitamin D. If you don't think you're getting enough calcium in your diet, consider taking calcium supplements. Antacids such as Tums are a good option, but remember to wait at least one hour after taking your thyroid hormone before taking calcium. You can supplement your vitamin D by taking two multivitamins (each with 400 IU of vitamin D) a day.

Another bone-boosting strategy is doing weight-bearing exercises three to five times a week, for twenty to thirty minutes at a time. It's also helpful to give up cigarette smoking and to drink alcoholic beverages in moderation. If necessary, you can take medications that help slow bone loss.

Heart Disease

Heart disease is the leading cause of death in the United States, accounting for 29 percent of all deaths in the country in 2001, according to the Centers for Disease Control and Prevention. Having hypo- or hyperthyroidism can make any pre-existing heart disease worse or put you at risk for heart problems that you don't normally have. Fortunately, prompt treatment can usually put a halt to these problems. But it's important to understand the risks of heart disease caused by thyroid disorders since heart disease is more prevalent among older adults.

Hypothyroidism affects the heart in several ways. It can cause elevated cholesterol levels in the blood by increasing the amount of cholesterol the body naturally produces in the liver. An underactive thyroid also increases the amount of cholesterol absorbed into the bloodstream and makes it harder for the liver to eliminate cholesterol.

Hypothyroidism also can cause hypertension or high blood pressure, which occurs when constricted blood vessels are forced to work harder to pump blood through the body. In people with hypothyroidism, the heart rate may be slowed significantly, which lowers the heart's ability to pump enough blood and causes hypertension. Having high blood pressure raises your risk for heart attack, heart failure, and stroke. The presence of high cholesterol compounds that risk.

Older people with hyperthyroidism may develop heart problems, too. Hyperthyroidism can cause abnormal heart rhythms, such as atrial fibrillations, which can worsen existing heart problems. Hyperthyroidism can also cause tachycardia, in which the heartbeat is rapid, at a rate above 100 beats per minute. In some cases, hyperthyroidism can bring about heart failure, in which the heart becomes damaged or is forced to work too hard. Anyone with underlying heart problems who develops hyperthyroidism is at greater risk for heart attack or stroke.

Myxedema Coma

Older adults who have suffered from untreated hypothyroidism for a long time are at risk for a rare life-threatening condition called myxedema coma. The condition may be triggered by a variety of factors, including infection, the use of certain drugs, severe stress, extremely cold temperatures, stroke, trauma, and heart failure.

When myxedema coma occurs, the patient's body temperature plummets, causing hypothermia. The patient may also experience delirium, a loss of lung function, a slowing of the heart rate, constipation, urine retention, stupor, and swelling. In addition, the condition causes the patient to become disoriented and suffer seizures. Eventually, the patient may fall into a coma and die.

⌶ Essential

Thanks to advances in medical care, which include better diagnostic tools and treatment, both myxedema coma and thyroid storm have become extremely rare. Nonetheless, they can occur and always should be treated as medical emergencies.

A myxedema coma is a medical emergency that warrants immediate attention and treatment. Treatment often involves intravenous injections of thyroid hormone. Because the condition can impair the body's ability to convert T4 into T3, patients are often treated with Cytomel (T3) as well. Unfortunately, death from myxedema coma is common, especially among older patients who have heart problems. The best treatment for myxedema coma is prevention, which means treating hypothyroidism before it becomes a serious problem.

Thyroid Storm

Elderly people who have hyperthyroidism are more likely to experience thyroid storm, a rare condition that affects a small percentage of people with an overactive thyroid. In people who have thyroid storm, the heart rate becomes uncontrollably fast, and blood pressure rises to extreme highs. Other symptoms include a high fever, shortness of breath, chest pain, confusion, weakness, and extreme nervousness and mood swings. Some people have nausea and vomiting as well as profuse sweating. In severe cases, the patient may fall into a coma.

Like myxedema coma, a thyroid storm is a medical emergency that needs immediate treatment. Untreated, thyroid storm can quickly progress to a stroke or heart attack. The condition usually requires treatment with high doses of antithyroid medications, followed by iodine-containing compounds and therapy for any underlying condition that may be causing or contributing to the problem.

In addition to untreated hyperthyroidism, thyroid storm is more likely in people who develop infections, changes in blood sugar, and severe emotional stress.

Treatment Concerns for Older Adults

Treating thyroid disease in older people is more challenging than it is in younger adults. For starters, many older adults are on other medications, making it more likely that there will be a drug interaction. Older adults may also wrestle with memory problems, which make it a challenge to ensure that they take their thyroid drugs consistently. In addition, some drugs seem to have a more powerful effect on older patients. In this section, we'll take a look at some particular concerns that affect older people with thyroid disease.

Beware Amiodarone

Amiodarone (Cordarone) is an antiarrhythmic medication used to treat life-threatening ventricular arrhythmias when other therapies have failed. The medication works by slowing the nerve impulses of the heart. Problem is, amiodarone can cause many problems with thyroid function, including hypo- or hyperthyroidism.

The primary problem with amiodarone is that it contains iodine. In people who have undetected Hashimoto's disease, the excess iodine can bring on symptoms of hypothyroidism. In other people, the medication seems to trigger the release of stored thyroid hormone, which causes hyperthyroidism.

Stopping the medication may seem like a logical option, but amiodarone is currently one of only two drugs that can treat ventricular arrhythmias in people who have heart failure. The other drugs that can help are beta-blockers. But if your heart hasn't responded to beta-blockers, then your only option may be amiodarone.

To keep you on amiodarone, your doctor may give you thyroid hormone replacement, beta-blockers, or other medications to help control your thyroid problem. Less commonly, you may need surgery to remove the thyroid and become hypothyroid to stay on amiodarone. Treatment will depend on the individual patient, the severity of the heart problem, and the challenges of the thyroid disease.

Start Low, Go Slow

When it comes to treating hypothyroidism in the elderly, it's best to start on a low dose of thyroid hormone replacement. Dosages may be as low as 12.5 or 25 micrograms. Subsequent increases, if necessary, should be equally slow and gradual to ensure that the medication doesn't affect your heart. It might also take longer for the medicine to have its full effect since these drugs tend to remain in the body longer in older people.

Bad Mixes

Older people take a disproportionately large number of medications and account for approximately 30 percent of all prescriptions sold in the United States, according to the U.S. Food and Drug Administration. That's because many older people have medical conditions that require ongoing maintenance, such as arthritis, high blood pressure, diabetes, and heart disease.

Alert

Older adults who have Alzheimer's may need help remembering to take their thyroid hormone medication. Some people may also stop complying with proper drug use. If someone you know is wrestling with Alzheimer's, take steps to make sure she still gets her thyroid medication.

When you add thyroid disease to the mix, it often means taking yet another medication. That's why older adults who develop thyroid disease should be extra vigilant about telling their doctors about existing medical conditions and the medications they take. Consuming levothyroxine with anticoagulants, for instance, can make the anticoagulant more potent. It can also render insulin less effective. You should also talk to your doctor or pharmacist about the impact of certain foods.

The Thyroid and Mental Health

Many factors can raise the risk of depression among older adults. Having a thyroid disease, especially hypothyroidism, is one of them. Other health conditions considered a risk for depression include diabetes, heart disease, stroke, cancer, Parkinson's disease, and Alzheimer's disease. Depression may also be a side effect of taking certain medications—or not taking medications. For instance, forgetting to take your thyroid hormone replacement drug for hypothyroidism can cause depression. In addition, depression in the elderly may also be caused by isolation, loneliness, and the death of a spouse.

It isn't always easy to spot depression in older adults. But symptoms are the same as they are in younger people and include:

- Persistent sad, anxious, or "empty" mood
- Feelings of hopelessness, pessimism
- Feelings of guilt, worthlessness, helplessness
- Loss of interest or pleasure in hobbies and activities that were once enjoyed, including sex
- Decreased energy, fatigue, being "slowed down"
- Difficulty concentrating, remembering, making decisions
- Insomnia, early-morning awakening, or oversleeping
- Appetite and/or weight loss or overeating and weight gain
- Thoughts of death or suicide; suicide attempts
- Restlessness, irritability

If the depression is linked to thyroid disease, prompt treatment can help relieve these symptoms and improve your mood. So if you or someone you know is suffering from depression, consider asking to have your thyroid checked, especially if you have a personal or family history of thyroid and/or autoimmune disease.

CHAPTER 18

Complications
of Thyroid Disease

As you know, thyroid disease can be easily treated and managed without any ensuing complications. But when the disease goes undetected, poorly treated, or wrongly diagnosed, it can lead to other health problems that are potentially life-threatening. In this chapter, we'll take a look at some of the biggest health risks that can occur with untreated thyroid disease, including heart disease, high cholesterol, high blood pressure, and others.

Diseases of the Heart

Heart disease is a simple term that encompasses several coronary conditions. It includes high cholesterol, high blood pressure, atherosclerosis, angina, stroke, heart failure, coronary artery disease, and heart attack. At the root of heart disease is the buildup of plaque in the arteries, which can occur as a result of high blood pressure and/or high cholesterol. As the arteries become clogged, they become increasingly narrow, making it harder and harder for the heart to pump blood through the body. The final result can be a heart attack, in which the blood supply via an artery to the heart is cut off, or a stroke, when blood going to the brain is disrupted.

Heart disease is the leading cause of death in the United States, for both men and women. It is a chronic problem that requires a great deal of medical treatment and maintenance. Although modern medicine provides myriad procedures that can open up narrowed heart arteries, the underlying disease remains, causing significant lifestyle changes and restrictions on activities you once enjoyed. In some people, heart disease eventually leads to disability or death.

Because thyroid hormone affects every cell in the body, a deficit or overabundance of it can have profound effects on the heart and provoke the onset of heart disease. Certain heart conditions become more likely if you are also dealing with thyroid disease.

High Cholesterol

Most people don't think of high cholesterol as a form of heart disease, but in reality, it is a serious condition that sets the stage for the arterial damage that leads to heart attack, stroke, and other types of cardiovascular disease. Cholesterol is a naturally occurring fatlike substance that has several important roles in the body. It assists in the production of hormones and cell membranes, aids in the digestion and absorption of fats, and helps promote the synthesis of vitamin D when the skin is exposed to sunlight.

Essential

Your body naturally manufactures cholesterol in the liver, but you also get cholesterol from the foods you eat. The most problematic foods aren't the ones high in cholesterol, such as shrimp, but rather the foods that are rich in saturated fat, such as whole milk, red meats, and cheese, and in trans-fatty acids, such as packaged cookies, snack foods, and baked goods.

The problem occurs when there is too much cholesterol in our bodies.

According to the AACE, about 98 million Americans have high cholesterol, which is defined as cholesterol levels above 200 mg/dL.

Hypothyroidism is the third most common cause of high cholesterol, right behind diet and genetics. Having hypothyroidism specifically increases LDL, low-density lipoproteins, or the bad cholesterol, which is responsible for the buildup of damaging plaque in the arteries.

The Thyroid Link

The connection between hypothyroidism and cholesterol is simple: Without enough thyroid hormone, metabolism slows, making it harder for the body to metabolize cholesterol. As a result, the cholesterol lingers in the blood, where it can cause plaque buildup in the blood vessels. According to the AACE, the average cholesterol level for people with an underactive thyroid is 250 mg/dL, which is much higher than what is considered healthy, which is below 200 mg/dL.

Why It's Bad

Having high cholesterol raises your risk for other forms of heart disease, which is already a risk in older adults and in people who are overweight. Fortunately, prompt and proper treatment for hypothyroidism reduces that risk. According to the AACE, patients whose TSH levels are restored to normal will show an estimated 20 to 30 percent reduction in their cholesterol levels.

High Blood Pressure

Every day, your heart beats about 100,000 times. Blood pressure refers to the force of blood against the artery walls whenever the heart beats. Its measurement is expressed as two numbers, one over the other. Systolic pressure, the number on top, is the pressure exerted when the heart beats. Diastolic pressure, the number on the bottom, is the pressure exerted when the heart relaxes between beats. Ideally, your blood pressure should be 120 mmHg over 80 mmHg or below.

It's normal for blood pressure to vary throughout the day. But when blood pressure stays high, you are said to have hypertension. High blood pressure is dangerous because it forces the heart to work too hard, which can harden the arteries.

Fact

High blood pressure brings more people to a doctor's office than any other medical condition, according to the National Institutes of Health. Simply cutting back these visits by 10 percent would save $478 million each year.

Approximately two-thirds of all adults over age sixty-five have high blood pressure, which is 140/90 mmHg or above. Pressures between 120/80 mmHg and 139/89 mmHg are called prehypertension, a sign that you're on your way to developing full-blown hypertension. One of the most frightening things about high blood pressure is the absence of symptoms. If you have it, you probably don't know it. The higher your blood pressure, and the longer you have it, the greater your risk for heart attack, stroke, and kidney problems.

The Thyroid Link

Both hypo- and hyperthyroidism can affect your blood pressure. Hypothyroidism can lower the heart rate to less than 60 beats per minute, which reduces the heart's pumping capacity and increases the stiffness of blood-vessel walls. The combination of these changes can cause high blood pressure. Anyone with chronic hypothyroidism should have her blood pressure checked regularly.

In hyperthyroidism, the body becomes more sensitive to the hormone adrenaline, which causes your heartbeat to go up. An elevated heart rate, in turn, can cause blood pressure to increase as well. In some cases, it may be just the systolic pressure that goes up.

Why It's Bad

Like high cholesterol, high blood pressure is a disease unto itself, but also a contributing risk factor for the development of heart disease. The condition has no warning signs or symptoms, but once it develops, it lasts a lifetime.

According to the National Institutes of Health, approximately 65 million American adults have high blood pressure—that's one in three adults. Although the condition often occurs as a consequence of aging, not everyone who gets older gets high blood pressure.

If you learn that you have a thyroid disease, make sure your doctor monitors your blood pressure. Although treatment for underlying thyroid disease usually can sometimes correct the problem, some people may need medication to reduce their blood pressure. Making the right lifestyle changes can also help lower your blood pressure. Losing excess weight (even ten pounds), getting more exercise, and eating a healthy low-sodium diet can all rein in your blood pressure.

Heart Failure

Carrying groceries leaves you winded. At night, you gasp for breath. Your shoes are snug because your feet are swollen. You shrug off the discomfort as the result of recent weight gain and advancing age, but you may actually have heart failure.

Heart failure is not a heart attack but is a life-threatening condition that occurs when your heart is damaged or forced to work too hard. As a result, the heart can't pump enough blood to the other organs. According to the American Heart Association, nearly 5 million Americans are living with heart failure, and 550,000 new patients are diagnosed each year. The condition is especially common among African Americans, who tend to get heart failure at an earlier age and are more likely to be hospitalized or die prematurely. In recent years, the incidence of heart failure has gone up, causing more than a million hospitalizations a year.

While most forms of heart disease occur predominantly in men, heart failure is an equal-opportunity condition that's evenly split between the genders. Among women over the age of seventy, one in ten will wind up with heart failure.

Unlike heart attack, which occurs more suddenly, heart failure develops over several years and gets worse over time. Clogged arteries caused by high-fat diets and inactivity, high blood pressure, diabetes, cigarette smoking, and previous heart attacks stress the heart and gradually reduce its ability to pump blood. Other causes include abnormal heart valves, diseases of the heart muscle, heart defects, severe anemia, hypo- and hyperthyroidism, and abnormal heart rhythms.

 Alert

People with heart failure need to watch their sodium intake. Sodium causes the body to hold on to fluids, which means the heart has to work even harder to pump the additional fluid. Too much sodium exacerbates the swelling. So be wary of canned soups, seasoning packets, snack foods, and fast foods, which all contain a lot of salt. Opt for low-salt seasonings and low- or no-salt canned foods and snacks instead. Even better, eat fresh fruits and vegetables.

The Thyroid Link

Hypothyroidism slows everything down, including your heartbeat. If you have heart failure and develop hypothyroidism, your heart condition will worsen. Without enough thyroid hormone, the heart can't speed up to compensate for the weakness caused by heart failure.

Treatment for hypothyroidism should be started immediately, but the effects may take several weeks to kick in. It may also take a while before you pin down the proper dosage. In the meantime, you can take measures to improve heart health by continuing to take other medications you take for heart conditions, such as high blood pressure medications, and make the necessary lifestyle changes. Tough as it may sound, that means getting some daily exercise, losing excess weight, controlling stress, and eating a healthy diet.

People who have hyperthyroidism may get an unusual type of heart failure called high output failure. In this condition, the heart is pumping so fast that it doesn't have time to fill up with blood, so it becomes incapable of pumping enough blood to the body. Unlike regular heart failure, the medication used for high output failure slows the heart's rapid pumping. Treating the underlying hyperthyroidism also improves high output failure.

Why It's Bad

At first, heart failure is largely an invisible condition. Your heart will compensate for its deficiencies by getting bigger and pumping faster. Over time, as your heart's pumping ability diminishes, the heart can no longer compensate. The result is typically shortness of breath, persistent fatigue, and swelling in your feet and legs as fluid builds up in your body. You may also develop a nagging cough, caused by a backup of fluid in the lungs. In some people, it may become difficult to lie flat on their back.

These days, medications and lifestyle changes—like losing weight, eating healthy, and quitting smoking—can often allow patients with heart failure to live for several years. But experts agree: the best way to treat heart failure is to prevent it in the first place.

Atrial Fibrillation (AF)

In some people, the rapid heartbeat caused by hyperthyroidism can lead to a dangerous condition called atrial fibrillation. AF is the most common abnormal rhythm of the heart. The problem originates in the atria, the two upper chambers of the heart, where the contractions dictate the amount of blood that gets pumped through your body.

In healthy people, the heart beats and pumps blood with regular rhythm, usually at a rate of about sixty beats per minute. Sometimes, like when you're exercising, it beats faster. Other times, during sleep for instance, it's considerably slower. But in healthy people, the interval between heartbeats is always the same, thanks to regular electrical discharges that travel through the heart and cause contractions. These impulses originate in the atria, then travel to the ventricles, where blood is pumped. We feel this steady pumping in our pulse.

In people with atrial fibrillation, these intervals become irregular because the electrical discharges have become uncoordinated and rapid. The abnormal impulses travel to the ventricles of the heart, causing them to beat irregularly.

 Alert

Caffeine, alcohol, and stress can all make atrial fibrillation (AF) worse. If you have AF, nix the morning java, skip the after-dinner drinks, and take steps to minimize your stress levels. You should also steer clear of over-the-counter cough and cold remedies that contain pseudo-ephedrine, which can stimulate the heart.

AF affects about 2.2 million Americans. Many factors can lead to AF. High blood pressure, thyroid disorders, heart disease, and alcoholism are just a few of the risk factors for AF. The risk for developing AF also goes up with age. Experts estimate that the condition affects 3 to 5 percent of people over the age of sixty-five.

Many people with AF have no symptoms and are unaware of the abnormality in their hearts. Those who do experience symptoms may feel palpitations. Other symptoms include dizziness, fainting, weakness, fatigue, shortness of breath, and angina, chest pain caused by reduced blood flow to the heart. These symptoms are the result of less blood being delivered through the body. In some cases, your first symptom is a stroke.

The Thyroid Link

AF can be the result of hyperthyroidism, which can set off the heart palpitations and a rapid heartbeat. If you have AF, you'll need more than just treatment to correct the thyroid problem. You'll also need medication to slow the rapid heart rate, such as beta-blockers or calcium-channel blockers, as well as anticoagulants to prevent clotting. Although rare, AF can also occur in people being treated for hypothyroidism who take too much thyroid hormone replacement.

Why It's Bad

In people who have AF, the atria may quiver, causing blood inside the atria to pool and clot. If a piece of a blood clot in the atria leaves the heart and becomes lodged in an artery in the brain, you will have a stroke. In fact, about 15 percent of strokes occur in people with AF. AF also increases your odds for heart failure.

Stroke

Having AF definitely increases your chances for having a stroke, a debilitating, even deadly event that occurs when blood clots go to the brain. Stroke occurs when a blood vessel leading to the brain is blocked by a clot or bursts, and the brain can't get the oxygen and nutrients it needs to function. As a result, that part of the brain starts to die, and you have a stroke. The most common cause of stroke is high blood pressure, which can cause a blood vessel to rupture.

Essential

According to the American Stroke Association, the prevalence of high blood pressure in African Americans in the United States is the highest in the world. That may explain why African Americans are more vulnerable to stroke and have almost twice the risk of strokes compared to whites.

Strokes can be divided up into three different types. Hemorrhagic stroke is the most serious form and occurs when a weakened blood vessel bursts.

An ischemic stroke occurs when a blood vessel in the brain develops a clot and disrupts the blood flow to the brain. A clot formed in a blood vessel in the brain is called a thrombus. One that forms elsewhere and travels to the brain is called an embolus. These blood clots often come from the atrium of the heart in people who have AF.

Some people may have what is called a transient ischemic attack (TIA), which is considered a mini-stroke. A TIA occurs when blood flow to the brain is cut off for a short period of time, often less then fifteen minutes. Although painless, a TIA is a serious signal that something is wrong.

The Thyroid Link

The link between stroke and the thyroid goes back to an increased risk for AF, which is a leading cause of stroke. That's why it's so important to get elevated levels of thyroid hormone under control and to tame any problems with your heart.

Why It's Bad

Having a stroke is a life-changing event. Every year, approximately 700,000 Americans suffer a stroke. As the third leading cause of death in the United States, stroke kills 157,000 people a year. Those who survive are at greater risk for another stroke and may also suffer a host of physical disabilities and difficulties. Muscles may involuntary contract and flex. Balance problems may make you vulnerable to hazardous falls. Some people are left to endure excruciating pain.

Other lasting effects of a stroke include difficulty speaking, hearing, and communicating. Some people may have problems swallowing. Others may have personality changes, and may suffer apathy, depression, and cognitive challenges.

Osteoporosis

Many people don't give much thought to their bones—until they break one. And the weaker your bones, the more likely they are to break. In people who have osteoporosis, the risk for fracture is even greater.

Osteoporosis occurs when the body doesn't make enough new bone, or when too much old bone is reabsorbed by the body. Sometimes, it's a combination of both problems. According to the

National Osteoporosis Foundation, millions of Americans are at risk for osteoporosis, which literally means "porous bones."

Question

Can swimming strengthen my bones?
Swimming may be great for cardiovascular health and a great way to reduce stress, but unfortunately, it does little to strengthen your bones. To strengthen bones, you need weight-bearing exercises, those that force your muscles to work against gravity. Examples include strength training, jogging, hiking, and rigorous walking.

Osteoporosis affects approximately 10 million Americans, 8 million of them women. Another 34 million adults are at risk for osteoporosis and may have a condition called osteopenia, which is low bone mass. The condition becomes more common in postmenopausal women, who have lost the protective effects of estrogen. In fact, after age fifty, half of all women will have an osteoporosis-related fall in their lifetime. But here's the catch: people who have osteoporosis don't know they do—until they slip, fall, and break a bone.

The Thyroid Link

Untreated or poorly controlled hyperthyroidism is a major risk factor for osteoporosis. In people with an overactive thyroid, the thyroid hormone stimulates osteoclasts, the cells that break down bone. At the same time, thyroid hormone has no effect on osteoblasts, which are the cells that build bone. The result is a deficit in bone. People who are taking too much thyroid hormone may be at risk for osteoporosis, too, which is why establishing the proper dose is so important. Patients who are taking the right dose do not have that risk.

Other factors can also raise your risk for osteoporosis. These risk factors include being thin or underweight, being Caucasian or Asian, not getting enough calcium or vitamin D, smoking cigarettes, drinking too much alcohol, and avoiding weight-bearing exercise. If you are at risk, ask your doctor for routine bone mineral density exams, which can help detect the onset of osteoporosis. Once detected, you may be given medications that slow the rate of bone loss.

Why It's Bad

A simple fall in someone with osteoporosis can be devastating, especially in older adults. Within a year after the fracture, 20 to 25 percent of elderly women will die, usually as a result of health problems caused by inactivity, such as blood clots. After a year, 40 percent can't walk independently. And 80 percent lose the ability to do basic activities such as grocery shopping.

Obesity

Look around. As a nation, we have become increasingly overweight. A few pounds here. A few pounds there. Next thing you know, you're tipping the scales with numbers you never dreamed you'd see.

Today, a whopping two-thirds of Americans are overweight, and one-third of the nation is obese. Perhaps most troubling of all, the numbers of overweight and obese children are also on the rise, a phenomenon that promises to push epidemic rates of diabetes, heart disease, and certain cancers well into the next generation.

Essential

Experts agree: the best way to lose weight is a combination of healthy eating and regular physical activity. A healthy diet plan should restrict high-calorie foods and limit portion sizes. And remember, slow and steady weight loss is more likely to endure than a diet that sheds the pounds rapidly.

Obesity is technically defined as having a BMI of 30 or more. (See Chapter 15 for more on BMI.) Being obese is not just about being overweight. People who are obese have extra amounts of fat on their bodies.

It would be easy if everyone could blame their thyroid or their genes for their excess weight. But the truth is obesity is most often a problem of inactivity and eating too much. Too much time spent in front of the television and computer, overlarge portions, and lack of time to prepare healthy meals and exercise are also contributors. Over time, these habits can result in steady increases in body weight, which can eventually lead to obesity.

The Thyroid Link

In people who have hypothyroidism, metabolism slows down. When that happens, you're more likely to gain weight (though often not enough to constitute obesity). Other problems that add to the weight gain include bloating, constipation, and fatigue, which can make it hard for you to pursue physical activities.

Research suggests that thyroid hormones may also be involved in the body's secretion of and ability to use leptin, a hormone involved in fat storage. In healthy people, leptin sends a signal to the brain to stop eating and that there is now enough fat stored. In people who are obese or overweight, the blood levels of leptin are actually higher than normal, but the brain can't receive the signals sent by leptin. Exactly how leptin is associated with thyroid disease, however, is unclear and a subject for research.

Why It's Bad

Obesity is harmful in many ways. For starters, it can take a serious toll on your quality of life. The most menial tasks can be physically exhausting. You may feel depressed, angry, and frustrated. Outings with friends may be fraught with embarrassment and shame. On the job, you may face discrimination, ostracism, and rejection by colleagues.

Obesity also raises your risk for serious health problems, including high blood pressure, high cholesterol, type 2 diabetes, and heart disease. It can lead to stroke and certain kinds of cancer. In people who have arthritis, obesity taxes the joints. It can also cause sleep apnea, which will perpetuate your fatigue. In addition, obesity can cause death. Experts estimate that obesity kills 300,000 people each year.

So, what can you do about it? The best defense against obesity is prevention. By adopting a healthy lifestyle that includes regular physical activity and good nutrition, most adults can stave off obesity and prevent the health problems associated with it. In terms of thyroid health, it means getting proper treatment and control of your thyroid disorder.

CHAPTER 19

Good Thyroid Nutrition

You are what you eat—or so they say. That's why it's so important to pay attention to your diet, especially if you have a chronic condition such as thyroid disease. The foods you choose can have a tremendous impact on the way you feel as well as how much weight you gain (or lose). This chapter offers some strategies for smart eating when you have thyroid disease.

Basic Nutrition

Eating well is one of the cornerstones of good health. But unfortunately, most American diets these days are far from optimal. Most are laden with high-fat convenience foods, excess sugar, and too many calories from large portions. To make matters worse, mealtimes for many people have become erratic and irregular, with too many meals eaten on the run.

The truth is, the foods you choose and the way you eat can make a huge difference in your health. On a day-to-day basis, they can affect the way you feel, how well you sleep, and how energetic you are. Over time, they can influence your likelihood to become overweight or obese, and your vulnerability to serious diseases. To help you make smarter choices, it helps to have a general understanding of basic nutrition.

Carbohydrates

Low-carb. High-carb. You hear a lot about carbohydrates these days. Carbohydrates are your body's primary source of energy and come in two forms: simple and complex. Simple carbs are those found naturally in fruits, vegetables, and milk as well as foods that contain refined sugars, which have been processed to extract the natural sucrose found in plants for a sweeter flavor.

Simple carbs break down rapidly, giving you a quick burst of energy. Healthy simple carbs include fruits, vegetables, and low-fat dairy products. Unhealthy simple carbs include cakes, cookies, crackers, sugary cereals, and snack foods. Rice, potatoes, and corn are also simple carbs that some recommend avoiding.

Complex carbohydrates are considered the healthier carbs, and are made up of starches and fiber found naturally in legumes, grains, and vegetables. Starch is found in the storage systems of plants such as wheat, oats, potatoes, beans, and lentils. In the body, starches break down into simple sugars, but do so more slowly than the simple carbs do.

Fiber, however, cannot be digested in the stomach and converted into simple sugars. That's because humans lack the enzyme required to break it down. Instead of being taken up by your body for energy, fiber is excreted, a fact that has made it a powerhouse in treating and relieving digestive disorders. A more lengthy discussion on fiber appears later in this chapter.

To maximize your health, eat a moderate amount of complex carbs, which will help keep cholesterol levels down and minimize weight gain. Limit simple carbs to fruits and vegetables, which supply other healthy nutrients. Try to cut back on your intake of carbs composed primarily of refined sugars. These include cakes, cookies, crackers, candy, ice cream, potato chips, sweetened sugars and juices, and most snack foods. Some people, like Dr. Friedman, believe in and practice a low-carbohydrate diet. He completely avoids all unhealthy simple carbs and also minimizes complex carbs. You should talk to your doctor about the best foods for you.

Protein
Foods rich in protein supply the body with the amino acids needed to build, repair, and maintain body tissues. When your body

doesn't get enough carbohydrates or fats, it turns to protein for energy. Protein is found in meat, eggs, legumes, seeds, nuts, soybeans, and tofu. Getting enough protein, which is generally not a problem in the American diet, ensures healthy muscle and tissues.

 Fact

Although protein has long been associated with muscle-building, it really doesn't build muscle strength or size by itself. Only by combining protein with strength training can there be any muscle building. But remember, any excess protein you eat is stored as fat and not burned as energy.

One of the best things about protein is that it helps you feel full, so that you are less likely to overeat. In people with hypo- or hyperthyroidism who have an increased appetite, protein may help calm the urge to eat and minimize any excess weight gain.

Fats

Fats have been demonized for our nation's weight problems. But in reality, fat is an essential nutrient, vital to the brain and nervous system. It is also the substance that lends cheesecake its smooth, creamy texture and makes macaroni and cheese so rich and tasty.

The problem with fat is its high caloric density. Unlike carbohydrates and protein, which supply four calories per gram, fat delivers a whopping nine calories per gram, making it the most concentrated form of energy. Fat comes in four basic forms:

Monounsaturated Fats

Monounsaturated fats that occur naturally in avocados and olive oil are the healthiest fats.

Unsaturated Fats

Polyunsaturated fats are liquids found in vegetable oils such as safflower, sunflower, and corn and are not as healthy as monounsaturated fats. However, omega-3 fatty acids found in fish are a healthy form of polyunsaturated fat.

Saturated Fats

These are the unhealthy fats that clog arteries and raise the risk of heart disease. These are solid at room temperature and come from meat, whole dairy foods, butter, and palm and coconut oils.

Trans-Fatty Acids

These fats are not found in nature, but rather are produced when oils are hydrogenated to make them solid at room temperature. These are found in all processed foods, such as breakfast cereals, frozen pancakes, potato chips, crackers, and cookies. They're also found in margarine and shortening.

The problem with fat occurs when you eat too much of it. The dense calories make it a fast and surefire way to gain weight. And too much of the unhealthy forms of fat can lead to health problems such as heart disease, diabetes, and certain cancers.

Vitamins and Minerals

Mother always said to take your vitamins, and she was right— vitamins and minerals supply the body with important substances that maximize our health and body functions. While vitamins and minerals do not supply the body with energy, they do help facilitate reactions that produce energy from the foods you eat.

Vitamin A, for instance, guards against infections, while vitamin D helps strengthen bones. And we already know that iodine, a mineral, is essential to the production of thyroid hormone.

When you have thyroid disease, certain minerals and foods play a bigger role in how you feel and how well your medications work. In the rest of this chapter, we'll zero in on specific nutritional factors that can affect your health and well-being.

Iodine

Iodine occurs naturally in seafood, seaweed, and kelp—namely plants and animals found in saltwater. The mineral is also found in milk, meat, spinach, and eggs. The bulk of it in the American diet, however, comes from iodized salt.

The recommended daily dietary allowance of iodine for adults is 150 mcg. In pregnant women, the amount goes up to 220 mcg. And in women who are breastfeeding, it increases to 290 mcg. But rest assured. Getting these amounts is relatively easy. All it takes to reach the RDA for adults is half a teaspoon of iodized salt.

Too Much Iodine

People who have healthy thyroids can eat as much as ten times more iodine than what's recommended and still be fine. But in people who have a thyroid problem, too much iodine is unhealthy. Excess iodine can actually inhibit the production of thyroid hormone, causing goiter and hypothyroidism. And if you already have hyperthyroidism, excess iodine can make your symptoms worse.

Too Little Iodine

The typical U.S. diet these days is rich in iodine. In fact, it's more apt to have too much iodine than it is to be in short supply. Since the 1920s, the nation has enjoyed a plentiful supply of iodized salt. Worldwide, however, the lack of iodine is a common problem, and it remains a massive public health issue on a global scale.

Alert

If you suffer from chronic diarrhea or an illness in which absorption is inhibited, you may have trouble absorbing iodine into your body. In that case, you should have regular thyroid function tests to make sure your body is taking up enough iodine.

But if you're on a low-sodium diet, you may be at risk for not getting enough iodine. Without enough iodine, your body cannot produce the thyroid hormone it needs, and you will be at risk for hypothyroidism and goiter.

Soy

Asian cultures have known about soy for years, but soy is a relatively new food to the American diet. In recent years, soy has emerged as a nutritional powerhouse, thanks to studies that have linked it to fighting disease. Isoflavones, substances found in soy, are said to help combat breast cancer, tame the hot flashes of menopause, limit the bone loss that occurs in postmenopausal women, and reduce your risk of heart disease by lowering cholesterol. In essence, soy acts as a phytoestrogen, or plant estrogen.

But a study in early 2006 in the journal *Circulation* offered a more humble view of this wonder bean. The study found that isoflavones had only a slight effect on lowering LDL, the bad cholesterol. The researchers also found no significant effects on HDL, the good cholesterol, triglycerides, and blood pressure.

In addition, soy had little effect on hot flashes and bone loss in postmenopausal women. They also found no evidence that soy could treat or prevent certain cancers, including breast cancer. But the researchers did not discount the benefits of certain soy products, which are high in protein, fiber, vitamins, and minerals.

Where Is Soy?

Soy is a bean found in foods as varied as tofu, tempeh, soy milk, soy sauce, and miso, a soybean paste. The excitement over soy has unleashed a tidal wave of new soy products, including soy burgers, soy shakes, and soy cereals. People also use tofu to make chili, lasagna, and desserts.

Troubles with Soy

In people who have hypothyroidism, too much soy can aggravate a thyroid problem. The isoflavones found in soy can increase TSH levels, causing an increase in thyroid hormone requirements and the potential for goiter. In women, excess soy can cause menstrual irregularities that may lead to infertility.

Soy can also inhibit absorption of thyroid medications. So if you like to eat soy, make sure you don't eat it around the same time you take your thyroid medication. Instead, you should wait at least four hours after taking your thyroid medication before eating anything that contains soy.

The Caffeine Factor

Every morning, you awaken feeling tired and sluggish until you get that morning cup of joe. If you're like many people, you need a jolt of caffeine to get you moving, be it a cup of coffee or tea. According to a study in 2004, 87 percent of adults and 76 percent of children have caffeine in their daily diets, which is higher than the 82 percent and 43 percent, respectively, found in 1977.

The fact is, caffeine is a drug, a legal stimulant found in numerous foods and medications that can have profound effects on the central nervous system. Over the years, caffeine has been accused of contributing to a host of diseases and conditions, but no link has ever been confirmed.

What we do know is that caffeine stimulates your body's production of adrenaline, one of the fight-or-flight hormones. Although the initial surge of adrenaline gives you an energy boost, its subsequent decline causes a crash that can trigger carb cravings and overeating. Caffeine also causes a temporary rise in blood pressure and more frequent urination, which can increase your excretion of calcium. In excess, caffeine can cause insomnia, anxiety, and heart palpitations.

Where's the Buzz?

Caffeine is found in a variety of foods, including coffee, tea, soft drinks, and chocolate. It is also found in energy drinks, caffeinated water, diet aids, cold remedies, and certain menstrual pain relievers.

Restrict Caffeine

People who have thyroid disease should be wary about consuming too much caffeine. In people who have hyperthyroidism, too much caffeine can exacerbate your symptoms and make you feel even more nervous, anxious, and jittery. It can also worsen any heart irregularities.

L. Essential

If you're trying to cut back on your caffeine intake, do it slowly, one cup at a time, one day at a time. Cutting down abruptly in people accustomed to several cups a day can cause headaches, drowsiness, and problems with concentration. You might also want to try substituting decaffeinated beverages or water for coffee.

If you have weight problems associated with hypothyroidism, you may be tempted to try diet aids that contain caffeine. Caffeine's stimulant effects do seem to temporarily enhance weight loss. But the effects on weight come with a price, namely anxiety, nervousness, and sleep problems. In turn, the lack of quality sleep can stimulate your appetite, which would sabotage any weight-loss efforts. The bottom line is this: try to consume as little caffeine as possible.

Goitrogens

In healthy people, eating an abundance of fruits and vegetables has been touted as a key way to keep diseases like heart disease, cancer, and diabetes at bay. Fruits and veggies are also celebrated as key components for healthy weight loss and management. But in people who have thyroid disease, too many of certain fruits and vegetables may have a negative effect.

These foods are known as goitrogens, a word derived from the term *goiter.* Goitrogens stimulate the formation of goiters. These foods block the effects of an enzyme called thyroid peroxidase, which is needed for the production of thyroid hormone.

Types of Goitrogens

Many cruciferous vegetables are goitrogens. These include broccoli, cauliflower, brussels sprouts, cabbage, turnips, and rutabagas. But other foods such as spinach, strawberries, radishes, peaches, millet, soy products, corn, sweet potatoes, carrots, peanuts, and walnuts are also considered goitrogens.

Limit Goitrogens

People who don't have thyroid disease can enjoy these foods without much concern, but in people with thyroid problems, these goitrogens are potentially problematic, especially if eaten in excess.

To suggest that you give up these healthy foods, however, seems counterintuitive to good health, considering all the nutrients that these foods contain. A better option is to eat these foods in moderation and at a relatively constant amount from one day to the next. You should also make sure to get your TSH tested regularly. Also, these foods are less harmful to people who have adequate iodine intake, making them less detrimental to people living in the United States.

Calcium

Unfortunately, most women today do not get enough calcium in their diet. They drink soda instead of milk, refuse to eat leafy green veggies, and don't bother with a supplement. In fact, the average American diet contains only about 500 to 750 mg of calcium.

Although most of the calcium in your body is in your bones, the mineral also helps muscles to contract, blood to clot, and your heart to beat. If you don't get enough in your diet, your body will take what it needs from your bones, which will cause your bones to become thin. That's why adequate calcium intake is so critical.

 Alert

> If you're concerned about bone health, cut back on alcohol. Consuming more than seven ounces of alcohol a week—the equivalent of one drink per day—reduces bone density. Because alcohol affects your balance and coordination, it raises the risk of falls and hip fractures. Alcohol is also high in empty calories—seven calories per gram.

This thinning of bone is exacerbated in women with hyperthyroidism, due to the stimulation of osteoclasts by the excess thyroid hormone.

Where's the Calcium?

Most of the calcium you get comes from your diet. Good sources of dietary calcium include low-fat milk, yogurt, and cheese. An eight-ounce glass of skim milk, for instance, provides 298 mg of calcium, while an eight-ounce serving of yogurt delivers 415 mg. An ounce of Swiss cheese provides 219 mg. You can also find calcium in fortified orange juice, canned fish with edible bones, leafy green vegetables, and tofu.

In addition, calcium is found in supplements and multivitamins. But most multivitamins do not have enough calcium to satisfy your daily needs.

Get Your Calcium

Women with thyroid disease need to pay special attention to their calcium intake, especially if they have hyperthyroidism. According to the National Institutes of Health, if you're over age fifty and taking estrogen, you need 1,000 mg of calcium per day. If you're over fifty and not taking estrogen, you need 1,500 mg a day. Women between the ages of twenty-five and fifty should get 1,000 mg a day.

Chances are, you won't satisfy your requirements, so most women need to take a supplement, too. When choosing a supplement, be sure to check the label for the amount of *elemental calcium* in it. To maximize absorption, take supplements with food or orange juice. If you take more than 750 mg of calcium supplements per day, take one dose in the morning and another before bedtime, since your body can absorb only so much calcium at a time.

The Importance of Fiber

As you probably recall, fiber is a component of complex carbohydrates. Because humans lack the enzyme required to break it down, fiber cannot be digested in the stomach and converted into simple sugars. Instead it acts as a gastrointestinal broom, a nutritional wonder food that can lower cholesterol; ensure regular bowel movements; and aid in the treatment of gastrointestinal conditions such as hemorrhoids, constipation, and diverticulitis.

Essential

If you're trying to eat more fiber-rich food, do it slowly. Too much at once can cause uncomfortable gas and bloating. And make sure you drink enough water with the fiber to help it move through your system without causing a disruption.

There are two types of fiber: soluble and insoluble. Soluble fiber dissolves in water, which reduces the time it takes to empty the stomach, and lowers cholesterol levels. Good sources include dried peas and beans, apples, and oats. Insoluble fiber—known as roughage—cannot dissolve in water but absorbs water. Insoluble fiber adds bulk to the stool and helps move food through the digestive tract, thereby preventing constipation, a problem for people with hypothyroidism.

Good sources of fiber include oatmeal, broccoli, legumes, Brussels sprouts, whole-wheat bread, green beans, and the skins of fruits.

Most foods rich in fiber are also loaded with other nutrients.

In people who are battling weight gain caused by thyroid disease, a diet rich in fiber can help promote weight loss by displacing unhealthy foods with healthy ones. It can also help relieve the constipation that comes with hypothyroidism. In addition, fiber binds bile acids, which are rich in cholesterol, thereby lowering cholesterol levels.

If you do increase your intake of fiber, make sure to keep tabs on your thyroid function with routine tests. A diet rich in fiber may decrease the amount of thyroid medication that your body absorbs

Selenium

Selenium is an essential trace mineral that occurs naturally in the soil. In the body, selenium is used to produce selenoproteins, which act as antioxidants with vitamin E to protect against cell damage that can lead to heart disease and cancer. Selenium also aids in cell growth and boosts immunity.

In terms of the thyroid, selenium helps convert T4 to T3. A deficiency of selenium might lead to a reduction in available thyroid hormone, causing hypothyroidism. Studies have shown that a deficit of selenium can cause goiters. Some experts believe that too much selenium may also cause thyroid problems, namely hypothyroidism.

Selenium deficiency is rare in the United States, though some studies have suggested that the soil here may not be as rich in selenium as once believed. Some people may have difficulty with absorption if they suffer from severe gastrointestinal illness. But the condition does occur elsewhere in the world, in places such as China, where the soil is not rich in selenium. In regions that also have iodine deficiency, a deficiency of selenium typically makes thyroid disorders even worse.

Sources of Selenium

Animals fed on foods grown in selenium-rich soil are a primary source of selenium in the United States. Selenium is also found in nuts, seeds, and grains that were grown in these types of soil. Selenium is readily available in the diet through numerous foods, including chicken, brown rice, eggs, whole-wheat bread, walnuts, seafood, and liver.

Do I Need a Supplement?

If you have a gastrointestinal disease that inhibits selenium absorption, you probably need selenium supplementation. One example is Crohn's disease, an inflammatory bowel disease that occurs in the small intestine. Selenium supplements have been shown to improve autoimmune thyroiditis. Studies in Germany found that selenium supplements reduced the amount of autoantibodies in the blood. Dr. Friedman recommends that patients on levothyroxine therapy take 200 mcg of selenium a day to aid in conversion of T4 to T3. Selenium supplements are sold in drugstores and health food stores for a reasonable price.

Iron

Iron is a critical trace mineral involved in producing healthy red blood cells. It's an essential part of hemoglobin, the substance in blood that carries oxygen from your lungs to all your other body cells. Without it, you develop anemia, or iron deficiency, which can cause fatigue and lightheadedness. Iron is also needed to convert T4 to T3. Severe iron deficiency results in a goiter.

In the United States, iron deficiency is quite common, especially among women. Women generally have smaller iron stores and also lose iron each month with menstruation. As a result, iron deficiency affects approximately 20 percent of all women, and about half of all pregnant women have it as well. Meanwhile, only about 3 percent of men are iron deficient. The condition is also caused by low iron intake, gastrointestinal bleeding associated with ulcers, and the use of aspirin or nonsteroidal anti-inflammatory drugs.

Before true anemia develops, patients with mild iron deficiency will have a low ferritin level, which measures iron stores. Studies in the *British Medical Journal* found that low ferritin levels, even without anemia, are often found in patients with fatigue, which will easily improve with iron treatments. Dr. Friedman recommends iron treatment in people with a ferritin level below 50 ng/mL (nanograms per milliliter). He recommends taking enough iron to boost the ferritin level above 70 ng/mL.

Because iron deficiency is so common, many people must take iron supplements to build up their iron level. Pregnant women must also ingest higher amounts of iron, usually in a prenatal vitamin.

 Alert

> People with hypothyroidism who take iron supplements must be careful not to take their thyroid hormone replacement at the same time. In fact, they should take their thyroid medication first and take their iron at least four hours later. Taken together, iron can inhibit absorption of the thyroid medication.

In some people, even the ingestion of iron-rich foods can interfere with the absorption of thyroid medication. For that reason, you should always look at the iron content on food labels. Certain foods are iron-fortified and high in iron. For example, one serving of multigrain Cheerios contains 100 percent of your daily value of iron.

While you shouldn't avoid taking iron or eating iron-rich foods, you may need to experiment to figure out which foods affect your symptoms of hypothyroidism. If you have a difficult time striking the right balance, consider talking to a registered dietitian or nutritionist about how to manage your iron intake along with your thyroid medication.

Chapter 20

Healthy Living with Thyroid Disease

Okay, now you're an expert on thyroid disease. But the key is knowing how to put all this information to good use and to actually live healthfully while dealing with a thyroid condition. In this chapter, you'll learn the golden rules of good living, even as you deal with your thyroid disorder. It can be done! As you read this chapter, keep in mind all that you've learned throughout the book.

Take Your Medications

Many people shudder at the notion of taking too many drugs, but when you have a thyroid condition, medications are essential. Without thyroid hormone replacement, your body cells can't function properly. And if you have hyperthyroidism, beta-blockers may be necessary to tame a rapid heartbeat. Once you take them for a while, you will experience the benefits of these drugs. The key to good medicine management is taking your drugs consistently and safely.

Be Patient

It can sometimes take a while for the effects of thyroid hormone replacement to kick in. In reality, the impact of these medications varies from one person to the next. For some people, the effects begin in just two weeks. For others, it might take six weeks before improvements are noticeable. It can also take months before you and your doctor pinpoint the best dosage.

Antithyroid drugs take time to work, too—sometimes several months. The drugs do not wipe out the excess hormone already produced before you started taking the medications. In the meantime, you'll still be dealing with the uncomfortable symptoms of both types of thyroid medications.

But be patient. Finding the best dose is a matter of trial and error. Remind yourself that at least you've been diagnosed and that relief is in sight. You will eventually find the right dosage.

Follow Safety Rules

Every drug has its own set of safety rules about storage, when to take it, and how to take it. Abiding by those rules, however, is your job.

Alert

If you have small children in the house, make sure to keep all drugs out of reach. A report by the Centers for Disease Control and Prevention found that 53,500 children under the age of four were treated in emergency rooms for swallowing drugs not intended for them. Avoid calling medication "candy," and discard unused pills in places your child can't get into. And make sure visitors keep drugs out of reach, too.

Before taking any medication, ask your doctor and pharmacist about side effects and potential interactions with foods and drugs. Then follow those rules, without exception. And remember to take your medication at the same time every day.

Get Regular Checkups

When you have a thyroid condition, routine visits to your doctor become more frequent, especially at first, when you're trying to pin down the right dosage of medication or to ascertain the cause of your symptoms. Make these doctor visits a priority.

The health of your thyroid is critical to your well-being.

Find a Doctor You Respect

One way to ensure that you see your doctor is to find one you like. Seek out the services of a doctor you like, respect, and trust.

While you may need the services of a distant specialist at some point, you should eventually find a doctor who is nearby and convenient to your home or office for your routine monitoring. Find the best doctor you can, regardless of insurance issues. Don't let monetary matters get in the way of good thyroid health.

Make Appointments in Advance

Rather than call for a follow-up appointment, book your next visit at the end of your current one. Bring your calendar to every visit—you know you'll have to come back soon anyway. That way, you'll be more apt to make the next appointment—and keep it, too.

Learn as Much as You Can

When it comes to your health, knowledge is empowering. Not only does learning about a disease teach you about the illness, but it also helps you to manage it, live with it, and, ultimately, triumph over the hurdles and obstacles it throws your way.

The fact that you've read this book and gotten this far shows that you are already in the process of educating yourself about thyroid disease. But remember, knowledge is ongoing, not static. Keeping abreast of developments in thyroid research may help provide answers to your questions about your own condition. It will also enable you to speak intelligently with your doctor about your concerns.

Books

Poring through books remains a tried-and-true method for learning about anything, and thyroid disease is no exception. Most large bookstores and libraries have well-stocked health sections, broken down by disease. Some people may even want to consider creating their own small reference library. But remember, books do get old, and the information in them does, too.

The Internet

A more up-to-date way of staying abreast of thyroid information is through the Internet. Web sites dedicated to thyroid health provide ample information about thyroid disease. And you can browse through medical journals on PubMed (*www.pubmed.gov*) for the most current research as well as older studies.

L. Essential

If you're intimidated by the Internet, consider taking a course to help you get started. If you'd still rather not get online, visit your local library and ask a librarian for help locating resources on the Internet. Some librarians are now trained specifically in doing health research.

You can also find online support groups, where you can meet other patients who are dealing with thyroid disorders. For more information, see the Appendix in the back of the book.

Make Energy for Exercise

As a nation, we've grown increasingly sedentary, leading lives dominated by television, computers, and cars. But anyone who is concerned about her health—and in particular, maintaining her weight—needs to make exercise a part of her life. In people who have thyroid disease and are struggling with weight, exercise is important for staving off weight gain. It is also beneficial in preventing major illnesses such as heart disease and diabetes, which can be more likely in people with thyroid disease. The key is to make exercise a routine and essential part of your life!

Do Something You Like

It sounds obvious, doesn't it? And yet many people get locked into doing activities they don't like just because they think they should. After a few months, they quit and resume their sedentary ways.

A better option is to start with an activity you enjoy—truly enjoy. If the idea of going to the gym makes you yawn, then stop going. If you can't stand pounding the pavement, then don't. Instead, experiment with other activities that may be different from your usual routine. For instance, if you enjoy nature, consider hiking. Or if you loved swimming as a child, consider a water aerobics class.

Doing an activity you enjoy will help you build the habit of exercise.

Make It a Priority

You brush your teeth every morning, eat your greens every day, and take a vitamin every night. That's where exercise belongs, too, as a top priority in your routine, especially if the rest of your life is sedentary.

So how do you get to that point? Start by writing it down on your calendar, along with your lunch dates, business meetings, and doctor appointments—just like any other important engagement.

Then do whatever it takes to reinforce the activity. Bring walking shoes to work if you can take a stroll during lunch. Sleep in your exercise attire, if you prefer a morning workout. Enlist a friend to join you at the gym if the camaraderie gets you there.

After a while, your workout time will be as big a part of your schedule as mealtime, bedtime, and your favorite TV show.

Even more reinforcing are the changes you'll start to notice. You'll have more energy, sleep better, and have more muscle tone. And for those who have also cut back their food intake, you'll notice that you've started dropping those extra pounds.

Eat as Healthily as Possible

Making healthy food choices is not a priority for most people. These days, most people are eating on the run, skipping meals, and grabbing whatever is convenient. When they finally do sit down for a meal, the tendency is to overeat. But for anyone with a chronic health condition, including thyroid disease, eating well should be a priority.

Smart Foods

Any food, eaten in moderation, can have a place in your diet, even the occasional birthday cake, candy bar, and morning doughnut. But the key to eating well is to make sure the bulk of your diet is made up of fruits, vegetables, whole-grain foods, low-fat dairy, and lean proteins. For more details on smart food choices, see Chapter 19.

Practice Mindful Eating

These days, most people rarely sit down for a leisurely meal. We eat on the run, in front of a television, at a fast-food restaurant, in the car, in bed for a midnight snack—always while doing something else. Because eating is not our primary activity, we eat unconsciously and do not focus our attention on our food.

 Fact

Our bodies are equipped with genes that prevent weight loss, rather than weight gain. This evolutionary development grew out of times when our early ancestors had to survive periods of famine, which they endured by storing fat during times of plenty. This is known as the "thrifty gene" hypothesis.

In contrast, most Europeans eat more fat and calorie-laden foods than their American counterparts. And yet there is much less obesity in Europe. One reason is that Europeans eat smaller portions. Another reason is that Europeans take the time to enjoy their meal, allowing ample time for satiety signals to work. They also drive less and do more walking and bicycling.

The act of focusing and eating slowly is called "mindful" eating. Our problem is not that we think about food too much, but rather we don't give enough thought to the food we are eating. Being more mindful or conscious of the food you eat will help you maintain your weight. Combined with exercise and good food choices, mindful eating can help spur weight loss. The following guidelines will show you how:

- **Savor your food.** Enjoy each bite. Look forward to your meals.
- **Eat three meals a day.** If you want to skip a meal, skip dinner, but do not make up for it with late-night snacks.
- **Eat only when hungry.** Stop eating when you're no longer hungry, not when you're full.
- **Restrict meals to your kitchen**, dining room, or lunch-room table.
- **Don't do anything else when eating**, except talking to your family and friends. Don't read, work on the computer, talk on the phone, or watch TV.
- **Eat slowly, chew slowly, and take small bites.** Put down your utensils between bites.
- **Put a small portion on your plate** and remove the serving platter/cooking dish back to the kitchen. Never eat directly from the common pot (it is also unsanitary).
- **Don't leave tempting food in front of you.** This is especially important at restaurants, where there is usually bread on the table. Ask for the bread to be removed.
- **Sip water between each bite.** This will fill you up and slow your eating.

Remember, it's not just what you eat, but how you eat that makes a difference in maintaining your weight.

Manage Your Stress

Everyone has stress. Whether it's the child who's anxious about an exam or the adult who's struggling to get through a tough job assignment, stress is a normal part of life. It's also not necessarily a bad thing. In small doses, stress can enhance our performance, help us persevere through an emergency, and push us toward higher goals. More important, stress can be essential to our survival.

The problem occurs when the stress is chronic. When you feel stressed out all the time, your health can be affected. For one thing, you might start eating poorly. Not only are you more likely to grab a doughnut than an apple, but you're also less likely to exercise, sleep well, and take care of yourself.

 Alert

Many people deal with stress by overeating, which can trigger unwanted weight gain. If that's your pattern, learn to identify the stressors and develop other, nonfood ways for coping, such as calling a friend, taking a walk, or writing in a journal. Make plans to do these things before the stress strikes.

If you have a chronic condition like thyroid disease, you may be less likely to remember your medications, make necessary doctor appointments, and take measures to stay well. And if stress evolves into full-blown depression, which it can, you may adopt a lackadaisical attitude that can interfere with your efforts to stay healthy. That's why learning to manage stress is so important to anyone with a chronic illness.

Minimize Stressful Events

It sounds easy enough, but many people set themselves up for stressful events. They spend time with people they despise, perform tasks they feel resentful doing, and get themselves involved in situations they find distressing.

Changing the way you do things and learning to avoid stressful situations and people can go a long way toward reducing your stress. For instance, if you hate being late for appointments, leave your house a little early. If you can't stand dinner with the in-laws every week, tell your spouse you'd like to come every other week. If you hate your boss, start looking for ways to change jobs. The idea is to identify your stressors and then take actions that make them a lesser part of your life. Sometimes, just taking action can provide relief from the stress, even if change doesn't follow.

Keep Your Perspective

Stress doesn't just come from the actual events that occur in your life. It's also the result of how you perceive an event. For instance, you might find it stressful to plan a vacation. But your best friend might view it as an opportunity to do some armchair traveling. Shifting your thinking to a less stressful mind-set can play a key role in taking control of stress.

Try altering the way you view stressful situations. Maybe you can't give your annoying sister a personality makeover. But you can change the way you think of her.

Try Relaxation Exercises

No matter what you do, you will never completely rid your life of stress. That's where relaxation exercises can help. Making time to relax can make a world of difference in how you feel, mentally, physically, even emotionally. Here are just a few ways to incorporate relaxation into your day.

- Take a break with a cup of hot herbal tea.
- Go for a short walk with a friend.
- Give meditation a try. Even five minutes of mindful breathing can be refreshing.
- Take a stretching break every hour or two.
- Call a friend who makes you laugh.
- Get a massage.

Get Your Sleep

A good night's rest is important to your overall health for numerous reasons. Without it, you're grumpy, tired, and less able to function. You're also more likely to forget things, overeat, and avoid exercise. But in today's busy 24/7 world, many people sacrifice sleep to get things done. Many others suffer from insomnia, which is difficulty falling asleep or staying asleep.

If you have a thyroid condition, getting a good night's rest is critical. Here are some suggestions from the National Sleep Foundation on how to ensure a good night's rest.

- Keep a regular schedule. Get up and go to bed at the same time every day, even on weekends. Resist the urge to sleep in on weekends, so you can establish and sustain a regular wake-sleep cycle.
- Create a relaxing bedtime routine. Whether you read, listen to music, or soak in a tub, a restful routine can set the stage and relieve the stress and anxiety that make it harder to get to sleep.
- Avoid stimulating activities before bed, such as paying bills, playing games, or solving problems.
- Make it comfortable. If your mattress is older than nine or ten years, it might be time to replace it with one that is comfortable and supportive. Spend fifteen minutes testing it out in the store before you buy.
- Limit light and noise. Keep your bedroom dark, and minimize noise. The exception might be a sound machine that produces white noise, which can lull some people to sleep.
- Use your bedroom only for sleep and intimacy. Leave your work in the office and the TV in the living room. Limiting activities in your bedroom will help you associate the room with sleep.
- Watch what you eat and drink. Don't eat in the two or three hours before bed. Limit fluids, so you don't awaken at night for visits to the bathroom.

- Try to exercise regularly. Regular physical activity can promote sleep. But try to do it at least three hours before bedtime. If you want to make it a part of your daily routine, the best time is in the morning.
- If you have trouble falling asleep, get plenty of sunlight in the morning and avoid sunlight in the late afternoon.
- Avoid alcohol and nicotine. Both substances can lead to poor sleep, especially when used close to bedtime. Although many people think of alcohol as a sedative, it actually causes nighttime awakenings and less restful sleep.
- If you can't sleep, get up. Try reading a dull book, folding laundry, or watching TV. When you start feeling tired, go back and try again.
- Don't take worries to bed. Before going to bed, write down your worries and make a to-do list for the next day. Then, set them aside and focus your attention on relaxing.

Poor sleep on a regular basis can actually cause several health problems such as high blood pressure, diabetes, and weight gain. So don't shrug off insomnia, daytime sleepiness, or any other sleep problem. Talk to a doctor if you routinely have problems getting to sleep. But remember, it is possible that trouble sleeping may be the result of hyperthyroidism or overtreatment of hypothyroidism.

Listen to Your Body

It's easy to forget you have a thyroid condition when a little pill taken once a day eliminates all the symptoms. But every once in a while, pause and take stock of your health and how you feel. Do you feel more tired than usual? Are you feeling at all depressed? Have you gained any weight? Have you noticed your heart beating more rapidly? Some people, like Margaret, say they can feel it when their thyroids are off:

After living with hypothyroidism for a decade, Margaret can tell when her thyroid medication needs a tweak. She may fatigue more easily after a workout on the treadmill. She may notice symptoms of depression setting in. And once, she felt her heart beating too rapidly, which told her she needed to lower her dosage. These days, she is her own best gauge of when she needs to adjust her medication. When she feels something, she just calls her doctor.

If you sense anything is awry, call your doctor immediately. Explain your situation and try to get an appointment as soon as possible. Quick action will help you avert any uncomfortable symptoms that may be heading your way. It will also ensure that you are taking the right dosage for your health.

Getting control of your thyroid disease can be as simple as taking a daily pill. But practicing good health habits on an ongoing basis will help ensure that you and your thyroid stay healthy.

Thyroid-related Organizations

American Association of Clinical Endocrinologists (AACE)
1000 Riverside Avenue, Suite 205
Jacksonville, FL 32204
(904) 353-7878
www.aace.com

American Foundation of Thyroid Patients
P.O. Box 4914
Odessa, TX 79760
www.thyroidfoundation.org

American Thyroid Association (ATA)
6066 Leesburg Pike, Suite 550
Falls Church, VA 22041
(703) 998-8890
E-mail: admin@thyroid.org
www.thyroid.org

The Endocrine Society
8401 Connecticut Avenue, Suite 900
Chevy Chase, MD 20815
(888) 363-6274 or (301) 941-0200
www.endo-society.org

The Hormone Foundation
8401 Connecticut Avenue, Suite 900
Chevy Chase, MD 20815-5817
(800) HORMONE
www.hormone.org

Light of Life Foundation
P.O. Box 163
Manalapan, NJ 07726
(877) LOL-NECK (565-6385)

E-mail: info@checkyourneck.com
www.checkyourneck.com

National Cancer Institute
NCI Public Inquiries Office
6116 Executive Boulevard
Room 3036A
Bethesda, MD 20892-8322
(800) 4-CANCER
www.cancer.gov

National Graves' Disease Foundation
P.O. Box 1969
Brevard, NC 28712
(904) 278-9482
E-mail: nancy@ngdf.org
www.ngdf.org

National Institutes of Health
9000 Rockville Pike
Bethesda, MD 20892
(301) 496-4000
E-mail: NIHinfo@od.nih.gov
www.nih.gov

Thyroid Cancer Survivors' Association, Inc.
P.O. Box 1545
New York, NY 10159-1545
(877) 588-7904
E-mail: thyca@thyca.org
www.thyca.org

Thyroid Federation International
797 Princess Street, Suite 304
Kingston, ON K7L 1G1
Canada
(613) 544-8364
E-mail: TFI@on.aibn.com
www.thyroid-fed.org

Books, Articles, and Web Sites

Books

Ain, Kenneth, and Rosenthal, Sara. *The Complete Thyroid Book*. (New York: McGraw-Hill, 2005).

Ditkoff, Beth Ann, and LoGerfo, Paul. *The Thyroid Guide*. (New York: Harper Perennial, 2000).

Duyff, Roberta Larson. *American Dietetic Association Complete Food and Nutrition Guide*. (Hoboken, NJ: John Wiley & Sons, 2002).

Fischer, Harry, and Yu, Winnie. *What to Do When the Doctor Says It's Rheumatoid Arthritis*. (Gloucester, MA: Fair Winds Press, 2005).

Rosenthal, Sara. *The Thyroid Sourcebook*. (Los Angeles: Lowell House, 1998).

Rubin, Alan L. *Thyroid for Dummies*. (New York: Hungry Minds, 2001).

Ruggieri, Paul. *A Simple Guide to Thyroid Disorders*. (Omaha, NE: Addicus Books, 2003).

Shomon, Mary J. *Living Well with Graves' Disease and Hyperthyroidism*. (New York: HarperCollins, 2005).

Shomon, Mary J. *Living Well with Hypothyroidism*. (New York: HarperCollins, 2005).

Shomon, Mary J. *The Thyroid Diet*. (New York: HarperCollins, 2004).

Smolin, Lori A., and Grosvenor, Mary B. *Nutrition Science and Applications.* (Orlando, FL: Saunders College Publishing, 1994).

Articles

Print Articles

Abrams, J. J., and Grundy, S.M. "Cholesterol metabolism in hypothyroidism and hyperthyroidism in man," *Journal of Lipid Research*, vol. 22 (1981): 323–338.

"American Association of Clinical Endocrinologists Medical Guidelines for clinical practice for the evaluation and treatment of hyperthyroidism and hypothyroidism," *Endocrine Practice*, vol. 8 (Nov.–Dec. 2002): 457–469.

Brender, E., et al. "Adrenal insufficiency," *Journal of the American Medical Association*, vol. 294 (Nov. 16, 2005): 2528.

Bunevicius, R., et al. "Effects of thyroxine as compared with thyroxine plus triiodothyronine in patients with hypothyroidism," *New England Journal of Medicine*, vol. 340 (Feb. 11, 1999): 424–429.

Canaris, G. J., et al. "The Colorado Thyroid Disease Prevalence Study," *Archives of Internal Medicine*, vol. 160 (Feb. 28, 2000): 526–534.

Carpenter, K. J. "A short history of nutritional science: Part 3 (1912–1944)," *Journal of Nutrition*, vol. 133 (Oct. 2003): 3023–3032.

Ericson, Gwen. "Early childhood surgery saves those with gene for thyroid cancer," Washington University in St. Louis, press release, Nov. 3, 2005.

Gärtner R., et al. "Selenium supplementation in patients with autoimmune thyroiditis decreases thyroid peroxidase antibodies concentrations," *Journal of Clinical Endocrinology & Metabolism*, vol. 87 (April 2002): 1687–1691.

Gärtner R., et al. "Selenium in the treatment of autoimmune thyroiditis," *Biofactors*, vol. 19 (2003): 165–170.

Hancock, S. L., et al. "Thyroid diseases after treatment of Hodgkin's disease," *New England Journal of Medicine*, vol. 325 (Aug. 29, 1991): 599–605.

Krassas, G. E. "Thyroid disease and female reproduction," Fertility and Sterility, vol. 74 (Dec. 2000): 1063–1070.

Kumar, Vijay, et al. "Lingual thyroid gland: Clinical evaluation and management," *Indian Journal of Pediatrics*, vol. 71 (2004): 1143.

Lee, A., et al. "Choice of breastfeeding and physicians' advice: A cohort study of women receiving propylthiouracil," Pediatrics, vol. 106 (July, 2000): 27–30.

Meadows, M. "Pregnancy and the drug dilemma," *FDA Consumer* (May–June 2001).

Mohandas, R., and Lal Gupta, K. "Managing thyroid dysfunction in the elderly: Answers to seven common questions," *Postgraduate Medicine*, vol. 113 (May 2003). 54-68, 100.

Momotani, N., et al. "Thyroid function in wholly breast-feeding infants whose mothers take high doses of propylthiouracil," *Clinical Endocrinology* (Oxf), vol. 53 (Aug. 2000): 177–181.

Murphy, Kate. "For thyroid hormones, how low is too low?" *The New York Times*, Nov. 8, 2005.

Padberg, S., et al. "One-year prophylactic treatment of euthyroid Hashimoto's thyroiditis patients with levothyroxine: Is there a benefit?" *Thyroid*, vol. 11 (March, 2001): 249–255.

Philippe, P., et al. "Antepartum dental radiography and infant low birth weight," *Journal of the American Medical Association*, vol. 291 (April 28, 2004): 1987–1993.

Pomerleau, M., et al. "Effects of exercise intensity on food intake and appetite in women," *American Journal of Clinical Nutrition*, vol. 80 (Nov. 2004): 1230–1236.

Robbins, J., and Schneider, A. B. "Thyroid cancer following exposure to radioactive iodine." *Reviews of Endocrine and Metabolic Disorders*, vol. 1 (April 2000): 197–203.

Skinner, M. A., et al. "Prophylactic thyroidectomy in multiple endocrine neoplasia type 2A," *New England Journal of Medicine*, vol. 353 (Sept. 2005): 1105–1113.

Surks, M. I., et al. "Subclinical thyroid disease," *Journal of the American Medical Association*, vol. 291 (Jan. 14, 2004): 228–238.

Surks, M. I. et al. "The thyrotropin reference range should remain unchanged," *The Journal of Clinical Endocrinology & Metabolism*, vol. 90 (Sept. 2005): 5489–5496.

Electronic Articles

Barclay, Laurie. "Ethanol ablation safe, effective for thyroid cystic nodules," Medscape, June 20, 2003. *www.medscape.com*

Berman, K. D., and Shrier, D. K. "Subclinical hyperthyroidism: Controversies in management," *American Family Physician*, vol. 65 (Feb. 1, 2002). *www.aafp.org*

Kim, M. I., and Ladenson, P. W. "Hypothyroidism in the elderly," Chap. 9 (July 9, 2004). *www.endotext.com*

"Recommendation Statement Screening for Thyroid Disease," U.S. Preventive Services Task Force (USPSTF). *www.ahrq.gov/clinic/3rduspstf/thyroid/thyrrs.htm*

Sacks, F. M., et al. "Soy protein, isoflavones, and cardiovascular health," an American Heart Association science advisory for professionals from the Nutrition Committee, *Circulation*, vol. 113 (Jan. 17, 2006). *www.circ.ahajournals.org*

"Society of Nuclear Medicine Procedure Guideline for Therapy of Thyroid Disease with Iodine-131 (Sodium Iodide) version 1.0," February 10, 2002. Society of Nuclear Medicine. *www.guideline.gov*

Web Sites

Thyroid-related Web Sites

American Association of Clinical
Endocrinologists (AACE)
www.aace.com

American Thyroid Association (ATA)
www.thyroid.org

ArmourThyroid.com
www.armourthyroid.com

EndocrineWeb.com
www.endocrineweb.com

GoodHormoneHealth
www.goodhormonehealth.com

Hormone Foundation
www.hormone.org

MyThyroid.Com
www.mythyroid.com

National Graves' Disease Foundation
www.ngdf.org

Thyroid Cancer Survivors'
Association, Inc.
www.thyca.org

Thyroid Disease at About.com
www.thyroid.about.com

Thyroid Foundation of America
www.tsh.org

Thyroid-Info.com
www.thyroid-info.com

Additional Web Sites

American Academy of
Family Physicians
www.familydoctor.org

American Autoimmune Related
Diseases Association
www.aarda.org

American Dietetic Association
www.eatright.org

American Heart Association
www.americanheart.org

American Psychological Association
www.apa.org

Centers for Disease Control
and Prevention
www.cdc.gov

CFIDS Association of America
www.cfids.org

Crohn's and Colitis
Foundation of America
www.ccfa.org

eMedicine.com
www.emedicine.com

Endotext.com
www.endotext.com

Gail Devers
www.gaildevers.com

HealthCentral.Com
www.healthcentral.com

Human Growth Foundation
www.hgfound.org

The International Council
for the Control of Iodine
Deficiency Disorders
http://indorgs.virginia.edu/iccidd

Irritable Bowel Self-Help Group
www.ibsgroup.org

Lab Tests Online
www.labtestsonline.org

Lucille Packard Children's
Hospital at Stanford University
www.lpch.org/index.html

The Lupus Foundation
www.lupus.org

The Magic Foundation
www.magicfoundation.org

MayoClinic.com
www.mayoclinic.com

MedicineNet
www.medicinenet.com

MedlinePlus
www.nlm.nih.gov/medlineplus

National Alopecia
Areata Foundation
www.naaf.org

National Cancer Institute
www.cancer.gov

National Institutes of Health
www.nih.gov

National Osteoporosis Foundation
www.nof.org

National Sleep Foundation
www.sleepfoundation.org

National Women's Health
Information Center
www.4women.gov

North American Menopause Society
www.menopause.org

Nutrition.Gov
www.nutrition.gov

Pituitary Network Association
www.pituitary.org

Sjogren's Syndrome Foundation
www.sjogrens.org

Synthroid
www.synthroid.com

University of Maryland
Medical Center
www.umm.edu

UptoDate
www.uptodate.com

U.S. Food and Drug Administration
www.fda.gov

WebMD
www.webmd.com

Weight Watchers
www.weightwatchers.com

Wrongdiagnosis.com
www.wrongdiagnosis.com

Index

(HCG), 20, 191, 200
Hypertension, 253–55
Hyperthyroidism, 87–104. *See also*
Graves' disease
  about, 11, 87
  aging and, 241–44
  apathetic, 242
  causes of, 18–19, 87–89
  children and, 231–33
  complications from, 103–4
  diagnosing, 94–102
  goiters and, 87–88, 92, 99, 133
  hypothyroidism and, 89
  mild (subclinical), 100, 243–44
  misdiagnoses, 101–2
  pregnancy and, 195, 199–202
  remission, 120
  symptoms, 18, 89–94, 174–75, 176, 231, 232, 242
Hyperthyroidism treatment, 105–20
antithyroid drugs, 110–13
  for children, 232–33
  drug options, 110–13, 114, 117–20
  drug side effects, 112–13
  importance of, 93–94, 102–3, 232
  in older people, 242–44
  options, 105–6
  in pregnancy, 200–201
  RAI, 105, 106–10
  surgery, 116–17
  taking drugs correctly, 114–15
Hypopituitarism, 164–68
Hypothalamus, 2, 3–4, 163
Hypothyroidism, 16–18, 41–56
  about, 11, 16, 41
  causes of, 17–18, 42, 226–27
  central, 165
  characteristics of, 16–17
  children and, 223–29, 230–31
  congenital, 223–29
  cretinism and, 228–29
  diagnosing, 24, 47–56, 224–25
  euthyroid sick syndrome vs., 22
  goiters and, 45, 133

  mild (subclinical), 18, 53, 193, 243–44
  in older people, 240–41
  pregnancy and, 17–18, 19, 197–99
  primary vs. central, 42
  risk factors, 42–43
  subacute thyroiditis and, 83
  symptoms, 16, 17, 24, 43–47, 174, 175, 176, 227–28, 240–41
  weight problems and. *See* Weight
Hypothyroidism treatment, 57–70, 198–99
  diet and, 66–67
  drug combination precautions, 67–69
  drug options, 57–62
  importance of, 56, 246
  in pregnancy, 198–99
  side effects and complications, 69–70
  taking drugs correctly, 62–65
Imitators, of thyroid disease, 22–23, 177–90
  CFIDS, 15, 181–82
  Cushing's syndrome, 184–86
  depression, 177–78
  diabetes/insulin resistance, 178–79
  fibromyalgia, 182–83
  GH deficiency, 190
  lupus, 183–84
  menopause, 189–90
  panic disorder, 186–87
  PCOS, 15, 180–81, 195
  sleep apnea, 187–88
  thyroid diagnosis errors and, 22–23
Infertility, 45, 194–95
Inflammatory bowel disease, 82
Insulin resistance, 178–79
Iodine
  causing thyroid disease, 18, 19, 42, 88–89
  consuming, 269–70
  goiters and, 132–33, 134
  radioactive (RAI) treatment, 105,

size/shape of, 1–2
Thyroid hormone
  antithyroid drugs plus, 111–12
  changes, effects of, 2
  functions/mechanics of, 6–9
  goiters and, 19, 133
  high levels, 2. *See also* Hyperthyroidism
  low levels, 2, 4. *See also* Hyperthyroidism
Thyroiditis. *See also* Hashimoto's thyroiditis
  children and, 233–34
  forms of, 82–86
Thyroidologists, 28. *See also* Doctors
Thyroid receptors (TR alpha and beta), 7
Thyroid-stimulating hormone (TSH), 4, 6, 8, 18, 19
  blood test/levels, 48–49, 53–54, 55–56, 74, 95–96, 97, 100–101, 125, 134, 139–40, 224
  cancer cells and, 156
  central hypothyroidism and, 165
  desiccated (natural), 61–62
  postpartum thyroiditis and, 204
  pregnancy and, 191–92, 193, 194, 197, 198, 206
  suppressing, 135–36, 141
  thyroid cancer and, 161
Thyroid storm, 104, 247–48
Thyrotropin-releasing hormone (TRH), 4
Thyroxine (T4), 6–7, 8, 22
  blood test/levels, 224
  blood tests/levels, 49–50, 53–54, 75, 100–101, 125
  desiccated (natural), 61–62
  pregnancy and, 191–92, 200
  synthetic, 58–59, 61
Thyroxine-binding globulin (TGB), 7, 192
Toxic adenomas, 138, 141–42. *See also* Nodules

Toxic multinodular goiters. *See* Goiters
Treatments. *See* Drugs; specific diseases
Triiodothyronine (T3), 6–7, 8, 22
  blood tests, 50–51, 53–54, 96, 100–101, 125
  desiccated (natural), 61–62
  drug side effects, 70
  pregnancy and, 191–92, 200
  synthetic, 59–60, 61
TSIs/TSAs, 125, 201
Type 1 diabetes, 77–78, 178–79
Ultrasound, 134, 139, 148
Vitamins and minerals, 268, 273–78
Vitiligo, 80
Web sites, 297–98
Weight, 26, 207–22. *See also* Diet/nutrition
  of babies, 227
  bad cravings and, 212–13
  basic facts about, 209–10
  BMI and, 210
  diagnostic/treatment challenges, 211–13
  exercise and, 214–19, 282–83, 289
  gaining (on purpose), 222
  gaining (thyroid causing), 26, 43–44, 211–12, 262–64
  hyperthyroidism and, 91
  hypothyroidism and, 26, 43–44
  losing (on purpose), 213–14
  losing (thyroid causing), 26, 91, 123, 222
  obesity, 262–64
  thyroid affects on, 207–9, 211–13